Temporary Boost, Lasting Effects: A Study on SNAP Benefits and WIC Participation Trends

Sandeep

First Printing, 2024

Table of Contents

Chapter 1. Introduction

According to the Food and Agriculture Organization of the United Nations (FAO), "Hunger and malnutrition are the biggest risks to health worldwide" (Food and Agriculture Organization of the United Nations [FAO], 2020). Detrimental effects of food insecurity on adults include physical health problems, such as general health condition (Vozoris & Tarasuk, 2003), bad health exams performance(Stuff et al., 2004), oral health problems (Muirhead et al., 2009), sleep problems (Ding et al., 2014), diabetes (Seligman et al., 2007).; and psychological problems, such as mental health problems (Heflin et al., 2005), depression (Casey et al., 2004). As for infants and children, detrimental effects of food insecurity include physical health problems, such as general health (Gundersen & Kreider, 2009), congenital disabilities (Carmichael et al., 2007), non-cognitive problems (Howard, 2011), asthma (Kirkpatrick, 2010), oral health (Chi, et al., 2014); and psychological problems such as depression (Melchior, 2012), aggression, anxiety (Whitaker et a., 2006), suicide ideation (McIntyre, 2013), behavior problems (Huang et al., 2010); academic performance (Alaimo et al., 2001), social skills (Jyoti et al., 2005)

Despite its economic strength, food insecurity is a serious concern in the U.S. According to the newest food insecurity reports by the United States Department of Agriculture (USDA), 13.7 million households, 10.5% of all US households were not food secure in 2019 (U.S. Department of Agriculture [USDA], Economic Research Service [ERS], 2020). The composition of food secure and food insecure households differs in demographic traits. Among the food secure households, about 67.64% are white, non-Hispanic households, 11.52% are black, non-Hispanic households, and 13.12% are Hispanic households; In contrast, among the food-insecure households, about 49.5% are white, non-Hispanic households, 23.04% are black, non-Hispanic households, and 20.63% are Hispanic households (USDA, ERS, 2020).

To decrease food insecurity in the U.S., the Federal government funds 15 food and nutrition assistance programs that cost $92.4 billion in 2019 (Tiehen, 2020). The main programs include Supplemental Nutrition Assistance Program (SNAP), Special Supplemental Nutrition Program for Women, Infants, and Children (WIC), National School Lunch Program (NSLP), and School Breakfast Program (SBP). SNAP is the largest program in the U.S. that delivers nutrition assistance to low-income and no-income households. While SNAP recipients receive cash in an account, they can only use the benefits of qualifying food purchases. This book purpose is to investigate the participation in and the impact of two of the largest nutrition assistance programs in the U.S., SNAP, and WIC.

In response to the economic downturn, the American Recovery and Reinvestment Act (AARA) in 2009 established an unprecedented rise in SNAP benefits. On average, the increase in 2009 is about $80 per month for a four-people household. Based on the thrifty plan, the estimated cost of food at home for a household of four people is about $510 per month, showing the increase is a significant amount of money to SNAP recipients. The ARRA set the benefits to expire in November 2013. In the second chapter, I investigate whether this increase and subsequent decrease in SNAP benefits influence the types of foods SNAP recipients to purchase and the sensitivity of food categories to income changes. With the data from the Consumer Expenditure Survey Diary portion, ranging from 2007 to 2015, I use a difference-in-difference experimental design to estimate the impact of SNAP benefit changes on food-at-home, vegetables, fruits, non-alcohol beverages, and other food category expenditures. I also estimate the impact of the benefit changes on the share of food-at-home expenditures for each food category. My model results provide evidence that the rise in SNAP benefits cause an increase in expenditures on food-at-home, fruits, vegetables, non-alcoholic beverages, and dairy relative to non-SNAP households. In 2013, the decrease in SNAP benefits led SNAP recipients to decrease sweets' expenditures and has no statistically significant impact on any other category.

Though similar in purpose to SNAP, WIC targets some of society's most vulnerable members – pregnant women, postpartum women, infants, and children up to five years old who experience nutrition risk. WIC recipients receive food, information about a healthy diet, and referrals for health care. Unfortunately, WIC enrollment has declined nationally from 2011 (63.5%) to 51.1% in 2017. And the coverage rate declined across all the WIC target groups: infants, children, and women (USDA, 2020b).

In the third chapter, I use administrative data from the Ohio Department of Health to study enrollment trends and benefit redemptions trends from 2015 to 2019. I study factors that correlate with participation and redemption rates, such as economic activity, geographic location (urban vs. rural counties), race or ethnicity, and family structure. I provide graphics that illustrate county-level variation in enrollment and redemption patterns affected by these factors and empirically test whether these factors are statistically significant.

In the fourth chapter, I use the same administrative data as in chapter 2 to investigate whether the length of time in the WIC program influences health outcomes for children. Specifically, I study the impact of enrollment duration in the WIC program on risk conditions in children and the children's age-based BMI percentile. I consider the time length that children are in WIC as a plausible source of exogenous variation since children rely on their parents or guardians to enroll them in WIC. To capture unobserved household characteristics that might correlate with WIC's length, I also use household fixed effects in my model. I find that the longer children are in the WIC program, the fewer the risk conditions reported in the clinic visit report. I also find that the BMI percentile increases when children (aged 2 to5) stay longer in WIC, regardless of where they fall in the BMI distribution.

Research in this book adds to the overall understanding of participant behavior in the SNAP and WIC programs and how WIC participation can affect health outcomes in children. Notably, this research shows the impact of food assistance programs has on the lives of beneficiaries. Furthermore, this research highlights the importance of enrolling those in need and improving services to fit the needs of participants better.

Chapter 2. The Impact of In-kind Food Benefit Changes on Consumption: Evidence from SNAP

2.1 Introduction

The Supplement Nutrition Assistance Program (SNAP) is one of the largest anti-poverty programs in the United States, aiming to provide low-income and no-income households sufficient food and nutrition when they do not have enough resources. Households receiving SNAP benefits can use them to consume certain food categories in eligible grocery stores.

In 2009, the American Recovery and Reinvestment Act (ARRA) increased benefit levels for the SNAP and expanded SNAP eligibility to release the impact during the Great Recession. On average, the increase in 2009 is about $80 per month for a household of four, while the thrifty plan for the cost of food at home for a family of four is about $510[1], showing the increase is a significant amount of money to SNAP recipients. And in 2013, the benefits decreased when the ARRA expired. Beatty and Tuttle (2015) examine the rise in SNAP benefits led SNAP recipients to increase their food-at-home expenditures. Kim (2016) find SNAP recipients also increase housing and transportation expenditures because of the rise of SNAP benefits in 2009. Bruich (2014) finds that each $1 of SNAP benefit cuts reduces about $0.37 in grocery store spending. However, previous research has not addressed whether this benefit change affected the types of foods households purchase.

[1] Retrieved from Food Plans of Official USDA in 2009: https://fns-prod.azureedge.net/sites/default/files/usda_food_plans_cost_of_food/CostofFoodMar09.pdf

One report from USDA shows that about 20 cents of each food purchase dollar of households were spent on desserts, sweetened drinks, candy, sugar and salty snacks, (Garasky et al., 2016). Generally, SNAP households are more likely to have a lower quality of diets because of the high cost of nutrient-rich food (Blumenthal et al., 2014). Adults and children in the US do not have enough fruits and vegetables, and they do eat too many foods with added sugar, fat, and salt (USDA, 2010). In this study, by SNAP benefits changes, I examine the effects of benefits change on expenditures on detailed food categories, and I estimate income elasticities for different food categories (out of SNAP benefit) for SNAP recipients. This study uses a difference-in-difference design to investigate about the impact of SNAP benefits rise on household expenditure on food-at-home, vegetables, fruits, sweets, and other food categories. Using Consumer Expenditure Survey (Diary) data, I confirm that SNAP recipients increase their food-at-home, fruits, vegetable, dairy, and non-alcohol beverage expenditure when SNAP benefits increase, compared to non-SNAP low-income households. After 2013, SNAP recipients decrease expenditures on dairy and sweets expenditure when the SNAP benefits decrease. However, there is no evidence that SNAP recipients change their allocation of food-at-home expenditures because of SNAP benefits change.

This paper illustrates the importance of my research question to nutrition policy. From the Consumer Expenditure Survey (CES) Dairy data, the food-at-home expenditure and expenditure on different food categories are collected. This study illustrates the food categories that added SNAP benefits and may provide some insights into the current policy discussion.

2.2 Background

In 2017, 11.8% of US households were not food secure at some time during the year, which is about 15.0 million households and 40 million people. [2] Food insecurity, defined by the USDA, refers to the condition that at times during the year, the households are not certain or not able to acquire enough food that meets the needs of all the family members because of insufficient financial resources or other resources for food. Food insecurity has been proved to be related to multiple poor health outcomes for both children and adults.

The SNAP, which was known as the Food Stamp Program before, is the largest program in the U.S. that gives nutrition assistance to low-income households. Several criteria determine the eligibility to participate, including gross income, net income, and asset level. Households receiving SNAP benefits can only use them to purchase certain food categories in eligible grocery stores. They cannot purchase alcohol, medicines, hot foods, or any nonfood items with SNAP benefits. [3]. In 2018, total SNAP benefits distributed in the US amount to were about 60.8 billion dollars, with an average benefit per person per month averaging $125.79. [4] An early estimate of SNAP benefits showed that for low-income households, the benefits from the SNAP account for about half of their food-at-home expenditure (Wilde et al., 2013).

---

[2] The data source: https://www.ers.usda.gov/topics/food-nutrition-assistance/food-security-in-the-us/key-statistics-graphics.aspx#foodsecure

[3] From what can SNAP buy: https://www.fns.usda.gov/snap/eligible-food-items

[4] Data resource: https://www.fns.usda.gov/pd/supplemental-nutrition-assistance-program-snap

2.3 Literature Review

Adults and children in the US do not take enough fruits and vegetables, and they do eat too many foods with added sugar, fat and salt (USDA, 2010). Generally, households in SNAP tend to have a lower quality of diets because of the high cost of nutrient-rich food (Blumenthal et al., 2014). One report conducted by the USDA in 2016 shows that in 2011, the second largest expenditure food category of SNAP households was sweetened beverages, which was the fifth for non-SNAP households. As for vegetables and fruits, the expenditure ranks of SNAP households got these items are both lower than that of non-SNAP households (Garasky et al., 2016). Besides, there is evidence showing that SNAP is related to obesity in women (Dinour et al., 2007). As a result, it is very important to understand about the composition of food basket that SNAP recipients purchase.

It is also important to learn about the effect of income change on food expenditure allocation of SNAP recipients. Many studies have summarized the food consumption on different food categories in responses to changes in income, however, the influence from in-kind income changes varies by food category for low-income SNAP households is not well established. In general, the intake of fruit, fruit juice and unprocessed red meat are found to increase along with income increases for both male and female individuals in high income Western countries (Muhammad et al., 2017). As for dairy products, Bergtold, Akobundu and Peterson (2004) found the demands for milk and cheese decrease when income increases, while Lechene (2000) estimates income elasticity of milk and cream is about 0.05. Income elasticities for nonalcohol beverages vary because sugar-sweetened beverages, fruit juice, tea and coffee all belong to this category. Okrent and Alston (2012) find that the elasticities of demand for nonalcoholic beverages are close to zero, while Muhammad et al (2017) estimate that for people in Western countries, they spend about $0.2 more on fruit juice for every $1 increase in income. Previous research shows heterogeneous associations between income and food consumption, such as demographics, food category, and income. (Muhammad et al, 2017). There are important impacts of income level on income elasticities at household level, the higher the income level is, the lower the level of elasticities (Femenia 2019). As for food benefits recipients, Lusk and Weaver (2017) conduct an experiment to identify the effect of in-kind benefits and cash on consumption for inframarginal and extramarginal consumers in a lunchroom meal setting, they find that the marginal propensity to consume soda out of cash is about $0.067 and that out of in-kind benefits is about $0.075. They also find that restrictions on fruits and vegetables for in-kind benefits makes extramarginal participants and non-fruit/vegetables consumers spend more on fruits and vegetables.

The impact of SNAP on consumption, food security, and health are broadly discussed in the literature. Nord et al. (2009) confirm the effects of SNAP on improving family food security problems. Research shows that the introduction of SNAP helps reducing the likelihood of food insecurity by 30% (Ratcliffe, McKernan, and Zhang 2011). Additional evidence confirms that participation in SNAP for six months was related to a decrease in food insecurity points for 5% to 10%, including households with food insecurity children (Mabli et al., 2013). The food stamps program reduces out-of-pocket food expenditure and rise overall food consumption (Hyones and Schazenbach, 2009). Furthermore, research shows that SNAP raises infants birth outcomes (Almond, Hoynes, and Schazenbach 2011) and children health outcomes (Kreider et al. 2009). Almond et al. (2011) show that pregnant women who use the SNAP three months before the delivery have higher birth weight, and the largest gains are at the lowest birth weights.

The consumption responses to SNAP are also discussed in a large literature, especially whether the impact of in-kind benefits from SNAP on food expenditure is the same as the effect from an equivalent amount of cash. The marginal propensity to consume (MPC) food out of SNAP and the marginal propensity to consume out of cash transfers are often used to make the comparison. The classical economy theory predicts that inframarginal households, defined as those who spend more than they receive in benefits on food, they would treat their in-kind benefits the same as an equivalent of cash (Whitmore, 2002). The majority of SNAP recipients are inframarginal households (Hoynes et al., 2014). As a result, the marginal propensity to consume food out of SNAP and out of cash should be similar for the majority of SNAP households.

A large number of previous observational studies supported this prediction. The randomization experiments were conducted to distribute food stamps benefits in check or voucher, and results showed that spending on food for people receiving voucher benefits was only 5% higher than people receiving cash benefits (Ohls et al., 1992). Breunig and Dasgupta in 2005 analyzed data from U.S. SNAP participants and found that there is no difference between the marginal propensity to consume food out of cash income and food stamps income for single households.

On the contrary, a large literature finds that the marginal propensity to consume food out of SNAP benefits is larger than cash, which can be explained by behavioral economic using mental accounting theory from (Thaler 1980). Mental accounting refers to the behavior of individuals to categorize their income based on the source, and similarly, they assign their expenditure into different income accounts (Rockenbach, 2004). SNAP households may categorize their SNAP benefits income in a specific income account because they can only be used to buy certain food, so their marginal propensity to consume food out of SNAP benefits are different from that out of cash.

Fraker (1990) summarized that the marginal propensity to consume food out of food stamps benefits is about 2 to 10 times higher than that out of cash after reviewing 17 earlier articles. However, most of this early research was criticized regarding participation in food stamps program as exogenous and only comparing food stamps participant with similar non-participants. Participation in food stamps program was found to be correlated with food-at-home consumption preference (Currie 2004), so that food stamps participants may have a higher marginal propensity to consume food than non-participants with similar demographic characteristics. In this comparison, the marginal propensity to consume food out of food stamps was overestimated. In a quasi-experimental design, Hoynes and Schanzenbach in 2009 estimated marginal propensity to consume food out of SNAP in-kind benefits is about 0.16, which is almost twice of the cash income, 0.09. Recently, Beatty and Tuttle in 2014 used the increase of SNAP benefits in 2009 to estimate marginal propensity to consume food-at-home out of SNAP. In 2009, the ARRA increased SNAP benefits level and expanded SNAP eligibility as a function to stabilize the U.S. economy during the Great Recession. For example, the SNAP benefits increased by $80 per month for four-people family after the ARRA. In Beatty and Tuttle (2014), the estimation was 0.48, which was also higher than the theory predicted. CR estimation of MPC food out of SNAP benefits is important.

While numerous literatures have estimated income elasticities for food demand, or the effect of SNAP on consumption, how the influence from SNAP benefit change varies by food category for low-income SNAP households is not well established. The estimates for different food categories for low-income households can provide information on how consumers react to in-kind benefit change and then have impacts on the policy insights.

In this chapter, I tried to estimate the impact of SNAP benefits change on household expenditure on food-at-home, vegetables (fresh), fruits (fresh), meat and eggs, dairy products, cereal, non-alcohol beverages, and sweets, and also find the impact on allocation of food-at-home expenditure, I also provide an estimate of income elasticity for various food categories.

2.4 Theoretical Model

The classical economic theory predicts that inframarginal households treat in-kind transfer no different than an equivalent cash transfer (Whitmore, 2002). A majority of

SNAP recipients are inframarginal households, who spend more on food than the benefits they receive (Hoynes et al., 2014).

Figure 1 and 2 provide the model of consumer choice of food and other goods expenditure under increase and decrease of SNAP benefits for inframarginal households based on the Southworth (1945) model. Figure 1 shows that, for inframarginal households, as the value of in-kind benefits increases from CF_1 to CF_2, their budget constraint shifts right from C_1 to C_2, allowing more food expenditure and more other goods expenditure. This model estimates that for inframarginal households, when they have more SNAP benefits, their food and non-food expenditure will both increase with the new budget constraint, however, the rise of food expenditure will be less than the dollar value of increase in SNAP benefits. Figure 2 shows that, for inframarginal households, as the value of in-kind benefits decreases from CF_1 to CF_2, their budget constraint shifts towards left from C_1 to C_2, allowing less food expenditure and less other goods expenditure.

Figure 1. Expenditure Changes of Inframarginal Households due to an Increase in SNAP Benefits

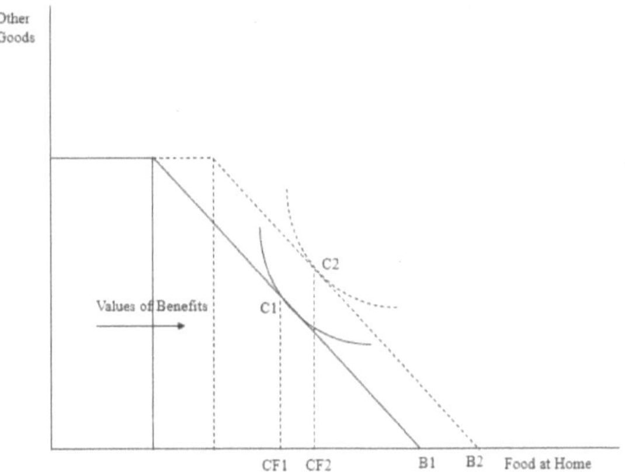

Figure 2. Expenditure Changes of Inframarginal Households due to a Decrease in SNAP Benefits

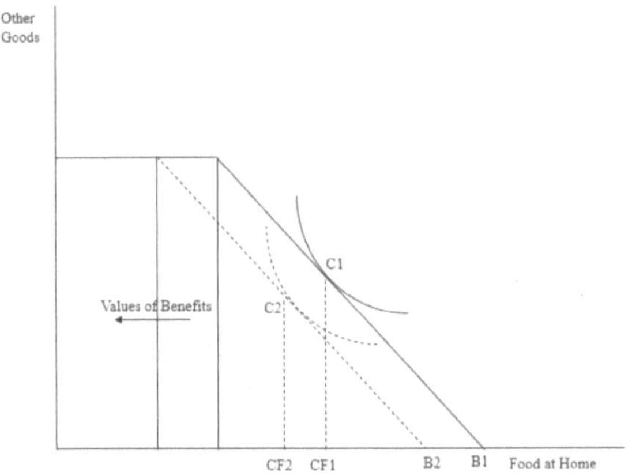

Figure 3 and 4 provide the model of consumer allocate a fixed budget to food at home and other goods expenditure under increase and decrease of SNAP benefits for

extramarginal households. Extramarginal households receive more SNAP benefits than their food budget, thus they have zero out-of-pocket expenditure on food-at-home, so their food expenditure budget equals to the SNAP value they receive. When they have more SNAP benefits, they will increase their food expenditure by the same amount as their SNAP benefits increase. Figure 3 shows that for extramarginal households, as their SNAP benefits rise from AF_1 to AF_2, their budget constraint shifts towards right from A_1 to A_2, keeping non-food expenditure the same. Figure 4 shows that for extramarginal households, as their SNAP benefits drop down from AF_1 to AF_2, their budget constraint shifts towards left from A_1 to A_2.

Figure 3. Expenditure Changes of Extramarginal Households due to an Increase in SNAP Benefits

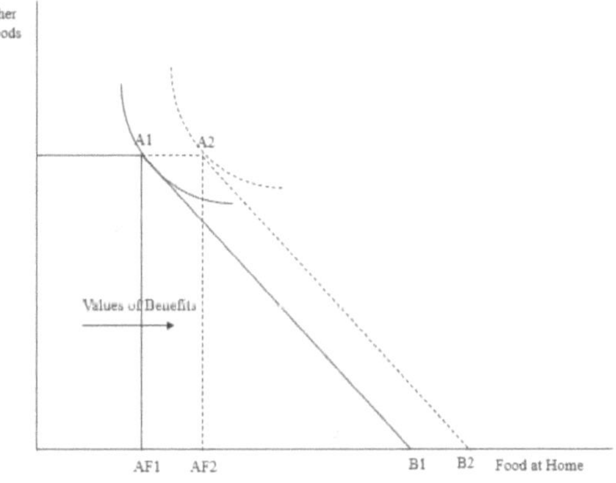

Figure 4. Expenditure Changes of Extramarginal Households due to a Decrease in SNAP Benefits

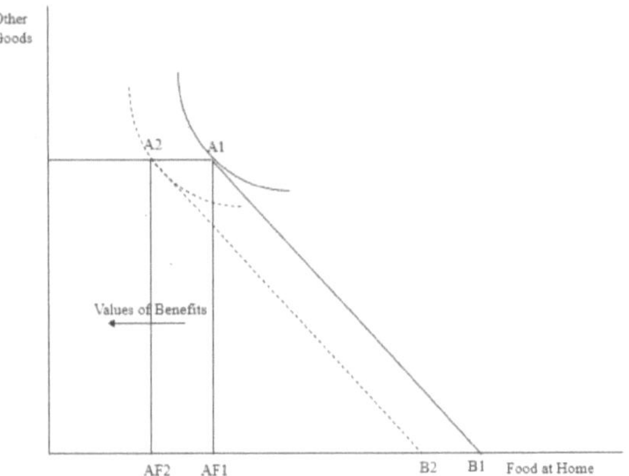

Table 1 shows the income elasticities of demand for aggregated food categories and significance tests from previous literature, Lechene (2000) and Muhammad et al. (2017). Lechene (2000) estimates income elasticities for both unaggregated and aggregated food products, some of the food products do not correspond exactly to the categories in this paper, so a range of elasticities are provided. Muhammad et al. (2017) estimate income elasticity of aggregated food products across region by age and by sex. Since the data I use in this paper is based on the expenditure of U.S. households, I select the estimates for western countries, and show the range of the estimates by sex and age.

Table 1. Income Elasticity Estimates of Key Food Categories with Previous Study

Food Category	Lechene (2000)	Muhammad et al. (2017)
Vegetables	0.09-0.27*	-0.07--0.02
Fruits	0.30*	0.05-0.17*
Dairy	0.05*	-0.00-0.04
Meat & eggs	-0.01-0.27*	-0.02-0.18*
Non-alcohol beverages	0.10-0.45*	-0.26-0.21*
Cereal	0.13-0.19*	-0.26--0.08
Sweets	0.00	na

*Designates statistical significance at the 10-percent level for estimates in previous studies Some of the food categories do not correspond directly to the categories in this paper, hence a range for multiple categories that corresponded to categories in this paper is showed.
Muhammad et al. (2017) presented income elasticities of food by gender and age, hence a range is generated here which include the max and min in previous research.

For vegetables, Lechene (2000) estimates a positive and significant income elasticities for both processed vegetables and fresh vegetables, but Muhammad et al, (2017) find negative and not significant estimates. For fruits, both of them confirm significant and positive income elasticities, ranging from 0.05 to 0.3. For dairy, Lechene (2000) provides a positive and significant income elasticity, which is about 0.5, for milk and cream, while Muhammad et al, (2017) estimates are all not significant for milk. For meat and eggs, Lechene (2000) finds positive and significant income elasticities for carcase meat and also meat products, and negative but not significant estimate for eggs, while Muhammad et al, (2017) find positive and significant income elasticities for unprocessed red meat but not significant elasticities for processed meat and fish. In Lechene's estimates, income elasticities for beverages (such as tea and instant coffee) are about 0.10, which is significant, income elasticity for fruit juices is about 0.45 and also significant. Muhammad et al, (2017) also find significant and positive income elasticities for fruit juice, which is about 0.20, but negative elasticities for sugar-sweetened beverages. As for cereal, Lechene (2000) finds positive and significant income elasticities for breakfast cereals and frozen convenience cereal foods, however, Muhammad et al, (2017) confirm negative, not significant elasticity for whole grains. Lastly, for sweets, Lechene (2000) estimates that the income elasticity is about 0.00 and not significant. And I do not find a directly or indirectly corresponding food category in Muhammad's work.

Based on the theoretical economic model, six hypotheses are made:

H1a: After SNAP benefits increase, inframarginal households increase their food-at-home expenditure.

H1b: After SNAP benefits increase, inframarginal households increase their expenditure in vegetables, fruits, dairy, meat and eggs, non-alcohol beverages, cereal and sweets.

H1c: After SNAP benefits increase, inframarginal households do not change their expenditure share in vegetables, fruits, dairy, meat and eggs, non-alcohol beverages, cereal and sweets.

H2a: After SNAP benefits decrease, inframarginal households decrease their food-at-home expenditure.

H2b: After SNAP benefits decrease, inframarginal households decrease their expenditure in vegetables, fruits, dairy, meat and eggs, non-alcohol beverages, cereal and sweets.

H2c: After SNAP benefits decrease, inframarginal households do not change their expenditure share in vegetables, fruits, dairy, meat and eggs, non-alcohol beverages, cereal and sweets.

2.5 Data and Methods

2.5.1 Data

The CES, which is collected by the U.S. Bureau of Labor Statistics (BLS), provides information on consumers expenditures for a variety of categories, income, and a host of demographic characteristics. The survey includes two distinct components: the interview and the diary survey. I use the diary survey for this study since it includes more detailed expenditures on foods participating households' purchase. I note that this survey is nationally representative and relies on a stratified sampling method. The CES represents the entire U.S. civilian noninstitutional population, which represents more than 98% of the U.S. total population. The sample of the CES survey include people living in apartments, houses, condominiums, and group quarters, such as dormitories in university, and it does not include military, people living in nursing homes, or people in prison.

In the diary survey, participating households navigate through several steps before they have completed the survey. First, they get interviewed by CES staff and provide information on household characteristics, income, and other important demographic traits. Then for two weeks households receive a booklet in which they enter, by hand, the items they buy and how much they spend. In these booklets households provide details on the types of food, clothing, and other expenditures they purchase. For example, in the food category a household might report how much its spends on apples, bread, cheese, cereal, milk, and restaurant visits. Readers can refer to Figure 5 (Gareau et al., 2013) for an example of a page in the diary. Once the two-week period has ended, CES staff collect the booklet back to the BLS where staff transcribe and include the data in the CES diary component. In this transcription, the BLS staff groups expenditures into categories and I provide a list of these general categories in Table 2.

Figure 5. Consumer Expenditure Survey Example of a Page in the Diary Survey

EXAMPLE | SUN MON TUE WED THU FRI SAT

1. Food and Drinks Away from Home

Examples: breakfast buffet, carry-out lunch, dinner & cocktails at restaurant, pizza delivery, Chinese takeout, child's school lunch, beer at happy hour, pretzels at ballgame, wine at tavern, croissant from café, ice cream from truck, wedding reception caterer, soda from vending machine, hot dog from convenience store, popcorn and soda at movies

Please unfold the LEFT FLAP to see Additional Examples

Level of detail needed: briefly describe the meal.

Include tax & tip for part 1 only.

Mark (X) one that best describes the type of meal: breakfast	lunch	dinner	snack/other	Description (See examples above and on the flap)	Mark (X) one that best describes where you made this purchase: Fast Food Take-out Delivery Concession	Full Service Places	Vending Machines or Mobile Vendors	Employer or School Cafeteria	Total Cost with tax & tip	If alcoholic beverages included, mark (X) all that apply: wine	beer	other	Enter the total cost of the alcohol
X				bagel, juice				X	2 79				
	X			pizza	X				5 57				
			X	coffee	X				1 35				
	X			sandwich, soda				X	5 15				
			X	chips			X		70				
	X			elem. school lunch - month				X	45 00				
			X	soda			X		65				
		X		buffet		X			62 23	X			12 00
			X	drinks from cash bar		X			15 00		X	X	15 00

Table 2. General Food Categories in Consumer Expenditure Survey Diary

<table>
<tr><td rowspan="19">Total Food</td><td rowspan="18">Food at home</td><td>Cereal and cereal products</td></tr>
<tr><td>Bakery products</td></tr>
<tr><td>Beef</td></tr>
<tr><td>Pork</td></tr>
<tr><td>Other meats</td></tr>
<tr><td>Poultry</td></tr>
<tr><td>Fish and seafood</td></tr>
<tr><td>Eggs</td></tr>
<tr><td>Fresh milk and cream</td></tr>
<tr><td>Other dairy products</td></tr>
<tr><td>Fresh fruits</td></tr>
<tr><td>Fresh vegetables</td></tr>
<tr><td>Processed fruits</td></tr>
<tr><td>Processed vegetables</td></tr>
<tr><td>Sugar and other sweets</td></tr>
<tr><td>Nonalcoholic beverages</td></tr>
<tr><td>Fats and oils</td></tr>
<tr><td>Miscellaneous foods</td></tr>
<tr><td colspan="2">Food away from home</td></tr>
</table>

The BLS then releases data on a quarterly basis. Households that participate in the diary survey also report participation in the SNAP program and the amount of SNAP money spent on food. Up until 2012, respondents answered two questions: 1) "Have any members of your CU received any Food Stamps, during the past 12 months?" 2) "Have any members of your CU received any Food Stamps, in the past month?" After each of these questions, the survey follows up by asking how much in SNAP benefits the household received. After 2012, the diary survey only asks the first of the two SNAP questions and the subsequent question about benefits. I describe how I manage this difference in survey questions below.

2.5.2 Sample Selection

For the purposes of my research, I rely on the CES diary survey from quarter 1 of 2007 through quarter 4 of 2015. This span of dates includes the benefit increase in April 2009 and the subsequent decrease in October 2013. For the benefit increase time frame, I use CES diary survey from quarter 1 of 2007 through quarter 4 of 2011. This sample time frame includes 37,076 total participants, and an average 1,854 each quarter. In the years when the survey asked both questions about SNAP participation and benefits, I observe 37,076 total responses to the first question and 4,731 responses to the second question, with average per-month benefits of $206.16. For this sample, I rely on the SNAP question that indicates participation in the last month, and only include those households that provide a dollar value for subsequent benefits question, which yields 34,875 respondents and an estimated SNAP participation rate of 7.36%. For the benefit decrease time frame, I use CES diary survey from quarter 1 of 2011 through quarter 4 of 2015. For this sample frame, I again keep SNAP households that answer affirmatively to the SNAP participation household and provide a benefit dollar amount, but for this sample, only the first SNAP question is considered, because the second SNAP question is not asked in the survey after 2012. This method results in 32,061 SNAP participants and an estimated participation rate of 9.91%. To make sure using one question to identify SNAP households works, I also use only one question to identify SNAP households for the SNAP benefits increase time frame and conducted the same regression analysis. The results are robust, and shown in Appendix Table 42.

The households in CES under report their SNAP participation, US estimates of SNAP participation in this time frame range from 9% to 15%, which are slightly higher compared to my estimates. In my analysis I divide the full sample into two smaller samples, one dedicated to the benefit increase and one dedicated to the benefit decrease. In the former sample, I have 9 quarters in the pre-increase period and 11 quarters in the post-increase period. For the later sample, I have 10 quarters in both the pre and post-decrease periods.

To create an appropriate sample, I first limit my sample to households with income on or below 200% poverty line. I choose this threshold because some states relaxed the poverty threshold for SNAP eligibility and households up to 200% of the poverty threshold can participate. This 200% of poverty threshold is also used as an eligibility constraint for TANF or other social benefits and households that are eligible for these benefits are automatically eligible for SNAP.[5] Broad-based categorical eligibility (BBCE) policy makes households become categorically eligible for SNAP, when they are qualified for Temporary Assistance for Needy Families (TANF) or State maintenance of effort (MOE). In the Table 3, I show all the States (43) that implement BBCE and the gross income limit of TANF/MOE program for each State.

---

[5] I also use 180% poverty-line and 150% poverty-line as threshold, and the regression results are pretty robust, the results are shown in Appendix Table 36-Table 39.

Table 3. States that Implement BBCE

State	Gross Income Limit of TANF/MOE Program[6]
Alabama	130%
Arizona	185%
California	200%
Colorado	200%
Connecticut	185%
Delaware	200%
District of Columbia	200%
Florida	200%
Georgia	130%
Guam	165%
Hawaii	200%
Idaho	130%
Illinois	165%
Indiana	130%
Iowa	160%
Kentucky	200%
Louisiana	130%
Maine	185%
Maryland	200%
Massachusetts	200%
Michigan	200%
Minnesota	165%
Montana	200%
Nebraska	130%
Nevada	200%
New Hampshire	185%
New Jersey	185%
New Mexico	165%
New York	200%/150%[7]
North Carolina	200%
North Dakota	200%
Ohio	130%

Continued

[6] This column shows the gross income limit of TANF for households without elderly or disabled members, and the income limits are presented as percentages of the Federal Poverty Guidelines (FPG)

[7] In New York, the gross income limit of TANF/MOE for households with dependent care expenses is 200%, for households with earned income, the income limit is 150%.

Table 3 Continued

Oklahoma	130%
Oregon	185%
Pennsylvania	160%
Rhode Island	185%
South Carolina	130%
Texas	165%
Vermont	185%
Washington	200%
West Virginia	200%
Wisconsin	200%

The table is referenced from USDA Broad-Based Categorical Eligibility updated on May 2020: https://www.cbpp.org/research/food-assistance/a-quick-guide-to-snap-eligibility-and-benefits#_ftn3

Since my intent is to investigate about the impact of the SNAP benefits changes on household food expenditures, I also limit my sample based on total reported expenditures for all households. First, I exclude 109 households (2007-2011) and 100 households (2011-2015) that report large total expenditures per person (top 1%) since these expenditures could include very large purchases, such as a car or large appliance, and consequently affect expenditures on other items at the margin. In the benefits increase time frame (2007-2011), the threshold is $3406.4 total expenditure per person in two-week long time period. In the benefits decrease time frame (2011-2015), the threshold is $4385.5 total expenditure per person for two-week long time period. I also remove households that report zero total expenditures during the two-week period. Households that report zero total expenditures may have been on vacation or experienced some other event and these would affect food expenditures in ways beyond the scope of my study.

Lastly, I restrict my sample of SNAP households to inframarginal households. These are households with total expenditures that exceed total SNAP benefits. For SNAP households, I select only inframarginal households that spend more on food than the benefits they receive. Since the expenditure data are in two-week intervals, I multiply total expenditures by 2 and compare this value to the reported value of SNAP benefits from the previous month. In my sample, 1,023 households are inframarginal in 2007-2011, 1,251 households are inframarginal in 2011-2015. I also verify reported SNAP benefits relative to amounts reported by USDA to make sure the household has reported an amount within the parameters of federal policy. [8]

I recognize the potential for respondents to self-select into the sample in general, and for those who are on the SNAP program to self-select to participate and to report SNAP participation and/or benefits. I report detailed demographic characteristics in Tables 2-4 for SNAP and non-SNAP recipients and emphasize that these summary statistics show minimal variation across quarters for the overall sample and for each sub-sample (SNAP and non-SNAP). I also show the detail demographic summary statistics of SNAP and non-SNAP households quarterly in Appendix Table 28 to 31. This limited variation suggests my sample has minimal sample selection bias.

Since the diary survey asks households to report details about expenditures over two weeks, I separate food expenditures into the following categories: a) all food; b) food away from home; c) food at home; d) all fruits; e) fresh fruits; f) all vegetables; g) fresh

---

[8] The maximum and minimum SNAP benefits are referenced from USDA Cost of Living Adjustment for each year: https://www.fns.usda.gov/snap/allotment/COLA

vegetables; h) meat and eggs; i) dairy; j) cereal; k) non-alcoholic beverages; and l) sweets. I also note that some households only reported expenditures for one week instead of two. In my analysis I rely on a two-week time frame so I assume that those who only report one week of expenditures would have spent the same amount in the second week and multiply their expenditures by two. In my sample, 9.12% only report one week of expenditures.

2.5.3 Summary Statistics

I report summary statistics for my sample in Tables 4, These tables include summary statistics for demographic characteristics and expenditures on food categories. In each case I report summary measures for the whole sample, then for the period of the benefit increase (2007-2011) and for the benefit decrease (2011-2015). The expenditures, income, and benefits received are all inflation adjusted, and the baseline inflation year is 2011. Demographic statistics reported in Table 4 show that overall, Caucasian respondents comprise 80% of the sample with African Americans comprising 15%. This distribution tends to vary with a higher proportion of African American respondents on SNAP and a lower proportion of Caucasians on SNAP. I also note that relative to the overall sample, respondents on SNAP more likely identify as female, have larger families, are younger, and have less education.

Average expenditures in Table 4 indicate that from 2007-2011, the average SNAP household spends nearly $205 on food at home in a two-week period. Non-SNAP households spend an average of nearly $122 in a two-week period. On average, SNAP household spend about $102.5 on food-at-home weekly, and non-SNAP households spend about $61 on food-at-home weekly. This difference in spending is in part due to the way in which I construct inframarginal households. Theoretically, food expenditures in inframarginal households exceed the SNAP benefits received, so by construction, none of the inframarginal households in my sample have zero expenditures, whereas some of the matched non-SNAP households have zero expenditures. Comparing with the summary statistics by USDA, in 2011 June, the average weekly cost of food at home for a family of 2 (aged between 19-50) with low-cost plan is about $107.60, with thrifty plan $84.5[9], SNAP households in my sample are between thrifty and low-cost plan, while non-SNAP households are lower than thrifty plan. This difference in expenditure between SNAP and non-SNAP households is common in the literature (Beatty & Tuttle, 2015). I also point out that expenditure shares are very similar between the two groups. Moreover, my difference-in-difference approach cancels out any time-invariant factors that might yield these differences.

In Table 4 I also show demographic characteristics of the 2011-2015 sample that I use to test the impact of the benefit decrease. Notably the 2007-2011 and 2011-2015 both include all four quarters of 2011. While the overall and non-SNAP household demographic characteristics are similar to those I observe in 2007-2011 sample, I do observe small differences in the distribution of race across SNAP households. In the latter sample I observe a higher proportion (75% compared to 69%) of whites and a lower proportion of African Americans (21% compared to 26%). Besides this small difference,

---

[9] Reference of data: https://fns-prod.azureedge.net/sites/default/files/CostofFoodJun2011.pdf

I observe similar patterns in race and expenditures between SNAP and non-SNAP households in this latter sample compared to the earlier sample.

Table 4. Summary Statistics for Benefit Increase (2007-2011) & Decrease (2011-2015)

	Increase (2007-2011)					
	Total		SNAP Participants		Non-SNAP	
Variable	Mean	Std.Dev.	Mean	Std.Dev.	Mean	Std.Dev.
White	0.80	0.40	0.69	0.46	0.82***	0.39
Black	0.15	0.35	0.26	0.44	0.13***	0.34
Asian	0.03	0.18	0.02	0.14	0.03**	0.18
Family size	2.36	1.61	2.81	1.79	2.30***	1.58
Age	51.22	20.08	46.83	16.92	51.79***	20.39
Single	0.41	0.49	0.30	0.46	0.42***	0.49
Female	0.61	0.49	0.73	0.45	0.59***	0.49
High School & Below	0.58	0.49	0.71	0.45	0.56***	0.50
Some college	0.30	0.46	0.24	0.43	0.30***	0.46
Bachelor & Above	0.13	0.33	0.05	0.23	0.14***	0.34
Last food stamps dollar value			206.16	164.26		
All Food ($US)	186.24	159.98	246.85	187.49	178.35***	154.32
Food away home ($US)	54.55	76.64	40.95	63.62	56.32***	78.01
Food-at-home (two weeks) ($US)	131.70	122.70	205.91	156.05	122.03***	114.18
All Fruits (two weeks) ($US)	11.98	14.90	16.32	18.26	11.41***	14.32
Fresh Fruits (two weeks) ($US)	7.90	11.44	10.12	13.07	7.61***	11.18
All Vegetables (two weeks) ($US)	11.81	14.47	16.98	17.26	11.14***	13.93
Fresh Vegetables (two weeks) ($US)	7.51	10.42	9.79	11.63	7.21***	10.21
Meat & Eggs(two weeks) ($US)	31.02	39.49	52.03	48.57	28.28***	37.29
Dairy (two weeks) ($US)	14.23	15.16	20.11	17.68	13.46***	14.62
Cereal (two weeks) ($US)	6.38	9.66	9.91	12.35	5.92***	9.15
Non-alcohol Beverage (two weeks) ($US)	12.58	16.13	20.42	20.28	11.56***	15.21
Sweets (two weeks) ($US)	4.67	8.18	7.35	10.52	4.32***	7.76
Total Expenditure Per Person (two weeks) ($US)	485.53	513.52	373.34	325.98	500.14***	531.39
Observations	8,430		979		7,420	
Share All Fruits of Food-at-home	0.09	0.09	0.08	0.08	0.09***	0.10
Share Fresh Fruits of Food-at-home	0.06	0.08	0.05	0.06	0.06***	0.08
Share All Vegetables of Food-at-home	0.09	0.08	0.08	0.06	0.09	0.09
Share Fresh Vegetables of Food-at-home	0.06	0.07	0.05	0.05	0.06**	0.07
Share Meat & Eggs of Food-at-home	0.21	0.16	0.25	0.14	0.21***	0.16
Share Dairy of Food-at-home	0.12	0.11	0.10	0.07	0.12***	0.11
Share Cereal of Food-at-home	0.05	0.07	0.05	0.04	0.05	0.07
Share Non-alcohol Beverage of Food-at-home	0.10	0.13	0.10	0.08	0.10	0.13
Share Sweets of Food-at-home	0.04	0.06	0.03	0.04	0.04	0.07

Continued

Continued Table 4

Observations	8,017		983		7,034	
	Decrease (2011-2015)					
	Total		SNAP Participants		Non-SNAP	
Variable	Mean	Std.Dev.	Mean	Std.Dev.	Mean	Std.Dev.
White	0.81	0.39	0.75	0.43	0.82***	0.38
Black	0.13	0.34	0.21	0.40	0.12***	0.33
Asian	0.04	0.20	0.03	0.16	0.05***	0.21
Family size	2.27	1.59	2.71	1.83	2.20***	1.54
Age	53.23	20.66	49.60	17.51	53.84***	21.08
Single	0.43	0.50	0.35	0.48	0.45***	0.50
Female	0.59	0.49	0.68	0.47	0.57***	0.49
High School & Below	0.54	0.50	0.64	0.48	0.53***	0.50
Some college	0.31	0.46	0.29	0.45	0.31	0.46
Bachelor & Above	0.15	0.36	0.07	0.26	0.16***	0.37
Last food stamps dollar value ($US)			209.69	166.40		
All Food ($US)	185.28	162.57	242.41	190.19	175.73***	155.46
Food away home ($US)	54.14	80.67	40.34	71.55	56.45***	81.88
Food-at-home (two weeks) ($US)	131.14	123.45	202.07	157.62	119.29***	112.51
All Fruits (two weeks) ($US)	12.41	15.97	17.02	19.75	11.64***	15.11
Fresh Fruits (two weeks) ($US)	8.62	12.46	11.18	14.84	8.19***	11.97
All Vegetables (two weeks) ($US)	12.38	15.08	18.16	18.21	11.41***	14.26
Fresh Vegetables (two weeks) ($US)	7.82	10.75	10.79	13.03	7.33***	10.24
Meat & Eggs (two weeks) ($US)	31.00	42.19	50.03	53.90	27.82***	39.01
Dairy (two weeks) ($US)	13.55	14.44	19.12	17.13	12.62***	13.72
Cereal (two weeks) ($US)	6.27	9.21	9.88	12.62	5.66***	8.36
Non-alcohol Beverage (two weeks) ($US)	12.73	16.94	20.72	24.60	11.39***	14.88
Sweets (two weeks) ($US)	4.64	7.88	7.06	10.29	4.23***	7.33
Total Expenditure Per Person (two weeks) ($US)	590.13	656.81	474.39	486.93	609.47***	679.18
Observations	8,142		1,214		6,928	
Share All Fruits of Food-at-home	0.09	0.10	0.08	0.07	0.10***	0.10
Share Fresh Fruits of Food-at-home	0.06	0.08	0.05	0.05	0.07***	0.08
Share All Vegetables of Food-at-home	0.09	0.08	0.09	0.07	0.09	0.08
Share Fresh Vegetables of Food-at-home	0.06	0.07	0.05	0.05	0.06**	0.07
Share Meat & Eggs of Food-at-home	0.22	0.16	0.24	0.14	0.21***	0.16
Share Dairy of Food-at-home	0.12	0.11	0.10	0.08	0.12***	0.11
Share Cereal of Food-at-home	0.05	0.07	0.05	0.05	0.05	0.07

Continued

Table 4 Continued

Share Non-alcohol Beverage of Food-at-home	0.11	0.13	0.10	0.09	0.11	0.14
Share Sweets of Food-at-home	0.04	0.07	0.04	0.05	0.04	0.07
Observations	7,745		1,214		6,531	

Note: Sample means are after matching. All the expenditures and benefits value are reported in 2011 dollars adjusted by the CPU Index. Statistical significant differences in means between SANP and non-SNAP are denoted by *** p<0.01, ** p<0.05, * p<0

In Tables 5-6 I show demographic characteristics and expenditures and expenditure shares for the two samples but separate the data into pre and post-policy periods. In Table 5, I report demographic characteristics and expenditures for the periods before and after the benefit increase. In this sample, I observe the increase in monthly benefits of nearly $40. I also observe an increase in both food at home and food away from home expenditures among SNAP households but no change among non-SNAP households. SNAP households also increase expenditures in each of the food categories I report, though large standard deviations and small magnitudes for the differences likely reveal these differences are statistically indistinguishable. For non-SNAP households, all differences are less than $2.00. This shows consistency across time in my non-treated group.

Table 5. Summary Statistics Before and After the Increase of SNAP Benefits(2007-2011)

	Before				After			
	SNAP Participants		Non SNAP		SNAP Participants		Non SNAP	
Variable	Mean	Std.Dev.	Mean	Std.Dev.	Mean	Std.Dev.	Mean	Std.Dev.
White	0.68	0.47	0.82***	0.39	0.70	0.46	0.82***	0.38
Black	0.27	0.45	0.13***	0.34	0.25	0.43	0.13***	0.34
Asian	0.01	0.11	0.04**	0.18	0.02	0.15	0.03	0.18
Family size	2.80	1.75	2.32***	1.59	2.82	1.81	2.29***	1.57
Age	46.03	16.99	51.74***	20.48	47.31	16.88	51.84***	20.31
Single	0.30	0.46	0.42***	0.49	0.29	0.46	0.42***	0.49
Female	0.72	0.45	0.59***	0.49	0.73	0.44	0.59***	0.49
High School & Below	0.74	0.44	0.57***	0.49	0.69	0.46	0.55***	0.50
Some college	0.20	0.40	0.30***	0.46	0.26	0.44	0.31***	0.46
Bachelor & Above	0.05	0.22	0.13***	0.33	0.05	0.23	0.14***	0.35
Last food stamps dollar value ($US)	183.94	144.14			219.56	174.02		
All Food ($US)	228.92	160.34	178.59***	150.44	257.66	201.45	178.15***	157.49
Food away home ($US)	37.12	58.01	56.37***	74.95	43.26	66.71	56.27***	80.47
Food-at-home (two weeks)	191.80	135.16	122.22***	112.78	214.40	166.93	121.88***	115.35
All Fruits (two weeks) ($US) ($US)	13.93	15.05	11.05***	13.32	17.76	19.82	11.72***	15.09
Fresh Fruits (two weeks) ($US)	8.56	11.98	7.24***	10.33	11.06	13.61	7.93***	11.84
All Vegetables (two weeks) ($US)	14.86	13.92	10.54***	13.22	18.26	18.89	11.64***	14.48
Fresh Vegetables (two weeks) ($US)	8.72	9.87	6.95***	9.96	10.44	12.53	7.43***	10.41
Meat & Eggs(two weeks) ($US)	49.75	47.80	28.63***	38.42	53.40	49.01	27.99***	36.33
Dairy (two weeks) ($US)	19.73	17.46	14.27***	15.13	20.34	17.82	12.79***	14.15
Cereal (two weeks) ($US)	9.21	13.49	6.00***	10.11	10.32	11.59	5.85***	8.26

Continued

Continued Table 5

Non-alcohol Beverage (two weeks) ($US)	18.97	17.63	11.84***	15.46	21.29	21.70	11.32***	15.00
Sweets (two weeks) ($US)	6.73	7.91	4.28***	7.97	7.72	11.81	4.35***	7.58
Total Expenditure Per Person (two weeks) ($US)	338.12	301.29	503.41***	535.66	394.57	338.46	497.42	527.86
Observations	377		3,375		606		4,072	
Share All Fruits of Food-at-home	0.08	0.09	0.09	0.09	0.08	0.07	0.10***	0.10
Share Fresh Fruits of Food-at-home	0.05	0.07	0.06	0.08	0.05	0.06	0.06***	0.08
Share All Vegetables of Food-at-home	0.08	0.06	0.08	0.08	0.09	0.06	0.09	0.09
Share Fresh Vegetables of Food-at-home	0.05	0.05	0.05	0.07	0.05	0.05	0.06***	0.07
Share Meat & Eggs of Food-at-home	0.25	0.14	0.21***	0.16	0.25	0.14	0.21***	0.16
Share Dairy of Food-at-home	0.11	0.07	0.13***	0.12	0.10	0.06	0.12***	0.11
Share Cereal of Food-at-home	0.05	0.04	0.05	0.07	0.05	0.04	0.05	0.07
Share Non-alcohol Beverage of Food-at-home	0.10	0.09	0.11	0.13	0.10	0.08	0.10	0.13
Share Sweets of Food-at-home	0.04	0.03	0.04	0.07	0.03	0.04	0.04	0.07
Observations	377		3,191		606		3,843	

Note: Sample means are after matching. All the expenditures and benefits value are reported in 2011 dollars adjusted by the CPU Index. Statistical significant differences in means between SANP and non-SNAP in before and after time period are denoted by *** p<0.01, ** p<0.05, * p<0.1

Table 6 reports demographic summary statistics and expenditures from pre and post periods relative to the SNAP benefits decrease. First, I notice a similar benefit amount ($223.35) in the period prior to the benefit decrease (2011-2015) relative to the benefit amount ($219.56) in the period after the benefit increase (2007-2011). On average, SNAP benefits decreased to $193.82 in the third quarter of 2013. For SNAP households, food at home expenditures fell as expected to a level very similar to expenditures prior to the 2009 benefit increase. I observe decrease in all food categories I report, but these magnitudes are small and may be statistically indistinguishable. For non-SNAP households, I observe minimal differences in expenditures before and after the benefit decrease.

Table 6. Summary Statistics Before and After the Decrease of SNAP Benefits(2011-2015)

	Before				After			
	SNAP Participants		Non SNAP		SNAP Participants		Non SNAP	
Variable	Mean	Std.Dev.	Mean	Std.Dev.	Mean	Std.Dev.	Mean	Std.Dev.
White	0.74	0.44	0.82***	0.38	0.76	0.42	0.82***	0.39
Black	0.22	0.41	0.12***	0.33	0.19	0.40	0.12***	0.33
Asian	0.03	0.16	0.04**	0.21	0.02	0.15	0.05**	0.21
Family size	2.78	1.91	2.18***	1.52	2.62	1.72	2.21***	1.57
Age	49.21	17.92	53.96***	21.03	50.06	17.02	53.70***	21.16
Single	0.35	0.48	0.45***	0.50	0.36	0.48	0.44***	0.50
Female	0.70	0.46	0.58***	0.49	0.67	0.47	0.56***	0.50
High School & Below	0.64	0.48	0.54***	0.50	0.63	0.48	0.51***	0.50
Some college	0.30	0.46	0.31	0.46	0.28	0.45	0.32**	0.47
Bachelor & Above	0.06	0.24	0.16***	0.36	0.09	0.29	0.17***	0.37
Last food stamps dollar value ($US)	223.35	174.78			193.82	154.73		
All Food ($US)	247.97	204.69	173.71***	151.74	235.95	171.75	178.27***	159.99
Food away home ($US)	39.44	73.51	55.32***	80.49	41.38	69.24	57.86***	83.57
Food-at-home (two weeks) ($US)	208.52	172.56	118.39***	108.77	194.57	138.02	120.41***	117.03
All Fruits (two weeks) ($US)	17.99	22.40	11.62***	14.58	15.90	16.09	11.65***	15.74
Fresh Fruits (two weeks) ($US)	11.54	16.48	8.14***	11.42	10.77	12.68	8.25***	12.62
All Vegetables (two weeks) ($US)	18.62	19.11	11.31***	13.66	17.64	17.11	11.54***	14.98
Fresh Vegetables (two weeks) ($US)	11.30	14.23	7.20***	9.55	10.20	11.47	7.48***	11.05
Meat & Eggs(two weeks) ($US)	50.73	51.91	26.89***	32.98	49.23	56.16	28.98***	45.42
Dairy (two weeks) ($US)	19.84	19.07	12.52***	13.31	18.27	14.54	12.74***	14.23
Cereal (two weeks) ($US)	10.12	11.49	5.82***	8.70	9.59	13.82	5.47***	7.92

Continued

Table 6 Continued

Non-alcohol Beverage (two weeks) ($US)	21.00	26.42	11.21***	14.29	20.39	22.32	11.62***	15.58
Sweets (two weeks) ($US)	7.66	12.02	4.30***	7.50	6.37	7.77	4.16***	7.10
Total Expenditure Per Person (two weeks) ($US)	502.61	524.11	678.72***	728.46	441.58	437.95	522.81***	600.93
Observations	675		3,829		539		3,099	
Share All Fruits of Food-at-home	0.08	0.07	0.10***	0.10	0.08	0.07	0.09***	0.10
Share Fresh Fruits of Food-at-home	0.05	0.05	0.07***	0.08	0.05	0.05	0.07***	0.09
Share All Vegetables of Food-at-home	0.09	0.07	0.09	0.08	0.09	0.07	0.09	0.09
Share Fresh Vegetables of Food-at-home	0.06	0.05	0.06	0.07	0.05	0.06	0.06	0.08
Share Meat & Eggs of Food-at-home	0.24	0.14	0.21***	0.16	0.24	0.15	0.21***	0.17
Share Dairy of Food-at-home	0.10	0.07	0.12***	0.11	0.11	0.08	0.12**	0.11
Share Cereal of Food-at-home	0.05	0.05	0.05	0.07	0.05	0.05	0.05	0.07
Share Non-alcohol Beverage of Food-at-home	0.10	0.09	0.11	0.14	0.11	0.09	0.11	0.14
Share Sweets of Food-at-home	0.04	0.04	0.04	0.07	0.04	0.05	0.04	0.07
Observations	674		3,626		539		2,905	

Note: Sample means are after matching. All the expenditures and benefits value are reported in 2011 dollars adjusted by the CPU Index. Statistical significant differences in means between SANP and non-SNAP in before and after time period are denoted by *** p<0.01, ** p<0.05, * p<0.1

2.6 Empirical Model

For the empirical methodology, I leverage the quasi-experimental design of the ARRA and focus on the change in SNAP benefits as a plausibly exogenous treatment effect. To estimate the (potentially) causal impact of SNAP benefit changes on food expenditures and expenditure shares I rely on a difference-in-difference (DID) estimation technique. With this estimation method I can control for a variety of factors, such as demographic characteristics and macroeconomic changes, which might affect my outcomes of interest. With this design I assume no pre-treatment trends and that both the treatment non-treatment groups would experience similar trends if the treatment had never happened (Angrist and Pischke, 2008). In Figures 6 and 7 I plot average quarterly expenditures for the whole sample and these figures show no indication of trends that could bias my estimates. To test this statistically, I regress each outcome variable on SNAP, time-trend, and the interaction of SNAP and time trend for before the policy change for both benefit increase and decrease time periods. In each case, the coefficient of the interaction is not statistically different from zero, except dairy expenditure before benefit increase, which means that the impact of benefit increase on dairy might not be accurate as other estimates.[10] In Appendix Figure 25 and 26, I plot the estimated average quarterly food at home expenditure before the benefits increase/decrease for both SNAP and non-SNAP households to show the parallel trend over time.

[10] The regression results for parallel trend assumption are shown in Appendix Table 40, 41.

Figure 6. The Mean of Food-at-home Consumption for SNAP and Non-SNAP Households from 2007 to 2011

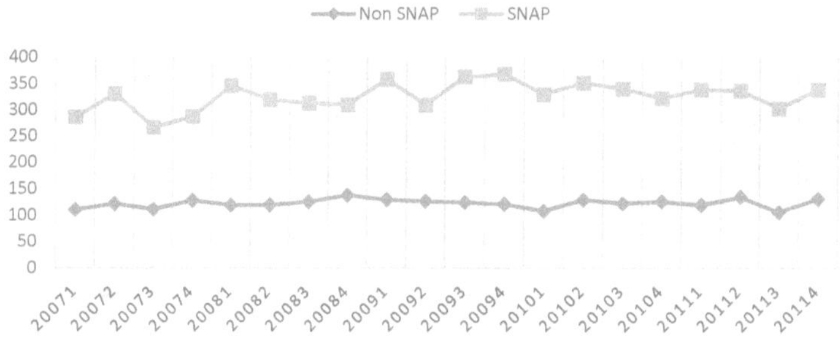

Figure 7. The Mean of Food-at-home Consumption for SNAP and Non-SNAP Households from 2011 to 2015

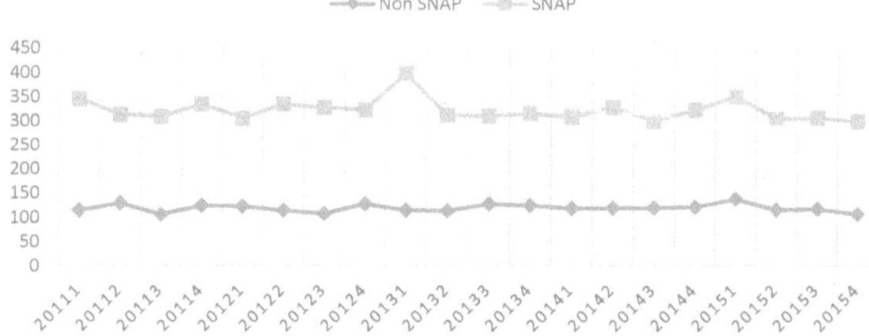

Since each quarter of data in the CES diary survey is a cross section of households I pool the relevant quarters together for my samples. To properly employ the DID method I construct a set of matched SNAP and non-SNAP households both before and after the benefit increase and subsequent decrease. This allows us to work with a pseudo-control group against which I can compare outcomes from those who receive SNAP benefits. For my matching method I utilize Coarsened Exact Matching (CEM) (Iacus, King and Porro, 2012) to increase the probability of getting matched households. With this method I coarsen the continuous variables household size and age by recoding them into categorical variables. I then match households based on these categories as well as race, marital status, employment, and the reported income group.

To estimate the effect of the benefit increase on food expenditures I rely on OLS regression based on the following model:

$$y_{itj} = \beta_{0j} + \beta_{1j}after_t + \beta_{2j}SNAP_i + \beta_{3j}after * SNAP + X_i\Gamma_j + \delta_t + v_t + \varepsilon_{ij}$$

Each y_{itj} represents a food expenditure or food expenditure share for individual *i* in quarter *t* for category *j* – food-at-home, vegetables, fresh vegetables, fruits, fresh fruits, dairy, meat and eggs, non-alcohol beverages, and sweets. The variable *after* is an indicator variable that has a value of 0 prior to the benefit change and a value of 1 thereafter. In the sample I use to study the benefit increase it has a value of 0 from the first quarter of 2007 to the first quarter of 2009 and 1 thereafter. In the sample I use to study the benefit decrease it has a value of 0 from the first quarter of 2011 to the second quarter of 2013, and a value of 1 thereafter. The variable *SNAP* is a dummy variable indicating whether household *j* has SNAP participants. The variable *after*SNAP* is the interaction term and its coefficient β_{3j} is the DID estimator and represents the average treatment effect on the treated (ATET). When I test the impact of the benefit increase on expenditures, my alternative hypothesis is $\beta_{3j} > 0$ to satisfy H1a-c. For the benefit decrease, my alternative hypothesis is $\beta_{3j} < 0$, to satisfy H2a-c. Last, I include a set of demographic controls, X_i, annual fixed effects, δ_t and quarter fixed effect, v_t.To account for heteroskedasticity in the errors, ε_{ij}, I estimate robust standard errors.

2.7 Results

2.7.1 Main Results

In Table 7 I present the main regression results of my analysis. Columns labeled 1 to 10 contain results for the different food categories I study. These results indicate that the SNAP benefit rise led participating households to increase food-at-home expenditures by an average of $20.37 ($p<0.05$) relative to non-SNAP households. Since I have expenditures for a two-week period, I multiply this point estimate by 2 and estimate that average monthly expenditures increase by $40.74, and this is very close to the increase in monthly benefits reported in Table 3. This is also close to the estimated increases in other related articles (Beatty&Tuttle, 2015). This result also indicates that I have sufficient evidence to support H1a.

Table 7. Main Results for SNAP Benefits Increase: 2007-2011

VARIABLES	(1) Food-at-home	(2) All Fruits	(3) Fresh Fruits	(4) All Vegetables	(5) Fresh Vegetables	(6) Meat & Eggs	(7) Dairy	(8) Cereal	(9) Non-alcohol Beverage	(10) Sweets
SNAP	59.05***	2.478***	1.167*	3.787***	1.659***	16.95***	4.582***	2.457***	5.863***	2.189***
	(6.825)	(0.786)	(0.615)	(0.703)	(0.509)	(2.483)	(0.861)	(0.910)	(1.060)	(0.430)
After	-14.87**	-0.596	-0.363	-0.718	-0.267	-3.446	-2.976***	-0.894*	-2.261**	-0.825*
	(6.460)	(0.782)	(0.573)	(0.794)	(0.586)	(2.187)	(0.938)	(0.524)	(0.956)	(0.469)
SNAP*After	20.37**	2.858***	1.567*	2.043**	1.042	3.801	1.857*	1.139	2.645*	0.805
	(9.213)	(1.097)	(0.813)	(1.022)	(0.710)	(3.118)	(1.080)	(1.006)	(1.376)	(0.645)
Observations	8,430	8,430	8,430	8,430	8,430	8,430	8,430	8,430	8,430	8,430
Demographic	YES	YES	YES	YES	YES	YES	YES	YES	YES	YES
Year and Quarter	YES	YES	YES	YES	YES	YES	YES	YES	YES	YES
Adjusted R-squared	0.257	0.132	0.110	0.144	0.115	0.174	0.196	0.120	0.132	0.0833

Notes: Regression include year and quarter fixed effects, control variables include age, single, employment, education, family size, race, income group. Robust standard errors in parentheses *** p<0.01, ** p<0.05, * p<0.1

They also consumer $2.86 more fruits (both fresh and processed), $2.04 more vegetables (both fresh and processed), $1.57 fresh fruits, $1.86 dairy and $2.65 more non-alcohol beverage, compared with nonparticipants when controlling for other variables because of policy changes. For the other food categories, the DID coefficients are not significant. In general, the model explained about 25.7% of the variance of food-at-home consumption. However, there is no evidence showing that SNAP participants change their meat and eggs, cereal or sweets consumption in response to the rise in SNAP benefits, my hypothesis 1b is partially supported.

Table 8 presents the main regression of Difference-in-Difference analysis for food-at-home allocations change when SNAP benefits increased, the regression coefficients and their standard error are included. Column 1 to 9 contain results for expenditure share in all vegetables (both fresh and processed), all fruits (both fresh and processed), fresh vegetables, fresh fruits, meat and eggs, dairy, cereal, non-alcohol beverage and sweets. From the results, I find no evidence showing that SNAP participants change their fruit, vegetables, meat and eggs, dairy, cereal, non-alcohol beverage or sweets allocations in response to increases in SNAP benefits, my hypothesis 1c is supported.

Table 8. Main Results for SNAP Benefits Increase: 2007-2011

VARIABLES	(1) Share All Fruits of Food-at-home	(2) Share Fresh Fruits of Food-at-home	(3) Share All Vegetables of Food-at-home	(4) Share Fresh Vegetables of Food-at-home	(5) Share Meat & Eggs of Food-at-home	(6) Share Dairy of Food-at-home	(7) Share Cereal of Food-at-home	(8) Share Non-alcohol Beverage of Food-at-home	(9) Share Sweets of Food-at-home
SNAP	-0.00470	-0.00525	-0.000729	-0.00360	0.0177**	-0.0181***	-0.00721**	-0.00514	-0.000579
	(0.00493)	(0.00379)	(0.00368)	(0.00296)	(0.00809)	(0.00454)	(0.00303)	(0.00547)	(0.00230)
After	0.00729	0.000608	0.00428	0.00591	-0.0124	-0.000618	-0.00933	-0.00421	0.00117
	(0.00575)	(0.00445)	(0.00535)	(0.00465)	(0.00990)	(0.00715)	(0.00602)	(0.00845)	(0.00412)
SNAP*After	-0.00356	-0.00136	-0.00176	-0.00239	0.00931	0.00200	0.00373	0.00191	-0.00305
	(0.00578)	(0.00446)	(0.00464)	(0.00364)	(0.00991)	(0.00533)	(0.00356)	(0.00662)	(0.00289)
Observations	8,017	8,017	8,017	8,017	8,017	8,017	8,017	8,017	8,017
R-squared	YES	YES	YES	YES	YES	YES	YES	YES	YES
Demographic	YES	YES	YES	YES	YES	YES	YES	YES	YES
Year and Quarter	0.0196	0.0272	0.0173	0.0204	0.0521	0.0205	0.0100	0.0215	0.00805
Adjusted R-squared	0.0172	0.0244	0.0141	0.0190	0.0512	0.0211	0.00992	0.0163	0.00849

Notes: Regression include year and quarter fixed effects, control variables include age, single, employment, education, family size, race, income group. Robust standard errors in parentheses *** p<0.01, ** p<0.05, * p<0.1

Table 9 presents the main regression of Difference-in-Difference analysis for expenditures change when SNAP benefits decreased, the regression coefficients and their standard error are included. Column 1 to 10 contain results for expenditures in food-at-home, all vegetables (both fresh and processed), all fruits (both fresh and processed), fresh vegetables, fresh fruits, meat and eggs, dairy, cereal, non-alcohol beverage and sweets. From the results, I find that on average, SNAP participants consume about $1.61 fewer sweets, compared to non-SNAP households after benefits decrease in a two-weeks long time period. However, for food-at-home and the rest of food categories, the DID coefficients are not statistically different from zero.

Table 10 presents the main regression of Difference-in-Difference analysis for food-at-home allocations change when SNAP benefits decreased, the regression coefficients and their standard error are included. Column 1 to 9 contain results for expenditure share in all vegetables (both fresh and processed), all fruits (both fresh and processed), fresh vegetables, fresh fruits meat and eggs, dairy, cereal, non-alcohol beverage and sweets. From the results, there is no evidence showing that SNAP participants change their fruits, vegetables, meat and eggs, dairy, cereal, non-alcohol beverage or sweets allocations in response to increases in SNAP benefits. The effect size of the regression coefficients of Did are shown in Appendix Table 32 to 35. The income elasticity for food-at-home and all the food categories are shown in Table 11.

Table 9. Main Results for SNAP Benefits Decrease: 2011-2015

VARIABLES	(1) Food-at-home	(2) All Fruits	(3) Fresh Fruits	(4) All Vegetables	(5) Fresh Vegetables	(6) Meat & Eggs	(7) Dairy	(8) Cereal	(9) Non-alcohol Beverage	(10) Sweets
SNAP	76.52***	5.190***	2.678***	6.000***	3.352***	18.25***	6.555***	3.264***	8.397***	3.252***
	(7.017)	(1.003)	(0.750)	(0.827)	(0.633)	(2.062)	(0.760)	(0.472)	(1.125)	(0.518)
After	-2.617	-0.136	-0.395	0.111	-0.407	0.118	-0.636	-0.0500	-0.256	-0.301
	(7.578)	(0.966)	(0.719)	(0.951)	(0.639)	(2.700)	(0.852)	(0.631)	(1.088)	(0.543)
SNAP*After	-13.12	-1.318	-0.392	-0.680	-1.078	-3.160	-1.686*	0.251	-0.834	-1.172*
	(8.753)	(1.199)	(0.920)	(1.099)	(0.802)	(3.093)	(0.961)	(0.760)	(1.488)	(0.617)
Observations	7,961	7,961	7,961	7,961	7,961	7,961	7,961	7,961	7,961	7,961
Demographic	YES	YES	YES	YES	YES	YES	YES	YES	YES	YES
Year and Quarter	YES	YES	YES	YES	YES	YES	YES	YES	YES	YES
Adjusted R-squared	0.264	0.127	0.112	0.154	0.132	0.171	0.194	0.133	0.130	0.0847

Notes: Regression include year and quarter fixed effects, control variables include age, single, employment, education, family size, race, income group. Robust standard errors in parentheses *** p<0.01, ** p<0.05, * p<0.1

46

Table 10. Main Results for SNAP Benefits Decrease: 2011-2015

VARIABLES	(1) Share All Fruits of Food-at-home	(2) Share Fresh Fruits of Food-at-home	(3) Share All Vegetables of Food-at-home	(4) Share Fresh Vegetables of Food-at-home	(5) Share Meat & Eggs of Food-at-home	(6) Share Dairy of Food-at-home	(7) Share Cereal of Food-at-home	(8) Share Non-alcohol Beverage of Food-at-home	(9) Share Sweets of Food-at-home
SNAP	-0.0134***	-0.0129***	0.00197	-2.11e-05	0.0141**	-0.0113***	-1.51e-05	-0.00830*	0.00143
	(0.00344)	(0.00275)	(0.00323)	(0.00261)	(0.00637)	(0.00381)	(0.00278)	(0.00486)	(0.00222)
After	-2.38e-05	-0.00249	0.00373	0.00204	0.00366	-0.000833	-0.00331	0.000544	-0.00150
	(0.00619)	(0.00496)	(0.00548)	(0.00453)	(0.0109)	(0.00653)	(0.00458)	(0.00964)	(0.00444)
SNAP*After	0.00522	0.00581	-0.000595	-0.00381	-0.00164	0.00211	-0.00222	0.00377	-0.000184
	(0.00483)	(0.00390)	(0.00468)	(0.00382)	(0.00934)	(0.00554)	(0.00369)	(0.00673)	(0.00333)
Observations	7,572	7,572	7,572	7,572	7,572	7,572	7,572	7,572	7,572
Demographic	YES	YES	YES	YES	YES	YES	YES	YES	YES
Year and Quarter	YES	YES	YES	YES	YES	YES	YES	YES	YES
Adjusted R-squared	0.0205	0.0239	0.0133	0.0232	0.0584	0.0167	0.00754	0.0109	0.0103

Notes: Regression include year and quarter fixed effects, control variables include age, single, employment, education, family size, race, income group. Robust standard errors in parentheses *** $p<0.01$, ** $p<0.05$, * $p<0.1$

47

Table 11. Income Elasticity of Food at Home and Aggregated Food Products

	Food-at-home	All Vegetables	All Fruits	Fresh Vegetables	Fresh Fruits	Meat & Eggs	Dairy	Cereal	Non-alcohol Beverage	Sweets
Income Increase	0.635	0.096	0.108	0.048	0.070	0.102	0.017	0.031	0.065	0.028
Income Decrease	0.473	0.033	0.071	0.037	0.026	0.051	0.053	0.018	0.021	0.044

48

2.7.2 Sensitivity

One of the key assumptions for the Difference-in-difference model is the parallel trends in dependent variable for control and treatment groups when policy has no change. To test whether SNAP and non-SNAP households experience semblable trends when SNAP benefits do not change, two placebo tests with the same specification strategy were conducted using only data after policy increase (2010-2011) and decrease (2014-2015). As shown in Appendix Table 43, there is no statistically significant coefficient on Did for food-at-home and all the food categories, as well as very small magnitude, which show that SNAP and non-SNAP households experience similar trends in those expenditures with the absent of policy change after the rise in SNAP benefits in 2010-2011. In Appendix Table 44, I find a statistically significant change of dairy at 0.1% significance level after the SNAP benefits decrease in 2014-2015, but no other significant results for food-at-home and the rest of food categories.

2.7.3 Limitations

I do not completely remove selection bias with the matching method – could still be an issue as long as unobservable characteristics exist that might influence participation in the program and food expenditures. Another limitation is how I construct bi-weekly expenditures. Over 90% of households include expenditures for both weeks, but for those that only report expenditures for one week, I multiply their expenditures by 2, and this maintains an assumption that expenditures in all categories are multiplied by 2, which may not be true. But I don't expect this to be a very serious problem in the results.

2.8 Conclusion & Discussion

In this Chapter, I investigate about the impact of increase and decrease in SNAP benefits on the expenditures of SNAP recipients. I find that SNAP recipients increase their expenditure on food-at-home, vegetables, fruits, dairy and non-alcohol beverage as a result of benefits increase. And these SNAP recipients do not change the allocation of their food-at-home expenditure because of the rise in SNAP benefits. Also, SNAP recipients decrease their expenditures on sweets as a result of SNAP benefits decrease. And they do not change their allocation of their food expenditure because of the cut in SNAP benefits.

This paper adds value to existing SNAP studies in two aspects. Firstly, I find out that SNAP benefit increase and decrease both affect expenditure on different food categories for SNAP households, which might be helpful for policy makers, especially when limiting food categories that SNAP benefit can purchase. Secondly, I figure out that SNAP benefit change do not lead to changes in the basket of foods SNAP households purchase.

Chapter 3 Analysis of WIC Enrollment and Redemption in Ohio

3.1 Introduction

In 2017, about 11.8% of US households were in food insecurity during some time of the year.[11] Many nutrition assistance programs distribute benefits to solve the food insecurity problem. In the fiscal year 2018, federal expenditures on 15 nutrition assistance programs surpassed $96 billion[12]. WIC is the third-largest nutrition assistance program, and it provides foods, referrals to health care, and nutrition education to low-income women, infants, and children who are at nutrition risk. In the fiscal year 2019, the cost of WIC by the Federal Government about $5.2 billion (USDA, 2020a). In April 2018, there were 7.8 million people enrolled in the WIC program (Kline et al., 2020). Among the participants, there were about 1.87 million infants, 4.15 million children under the age of 5, and 1.81 million pregnant, breastfeeding, and postpartum women[13].

Evidence shows that only 51.1% of eligible people (14.1 million) enrolled in WIC in 2017. This includes 79.3% of eligible infants, 41.8% of eligible children (aged 1 to 4), and 57.4% of eligible pregnant and postpartum women (USDA 2020b). WIC program

---

[11] The data source: https://www.ers.usda.gov/topics/food-nutrition-assistance/food-security-in-the-us/key-statistics-graphics.aspx#foodsecure
[12] The data source: https://www.ers.usda.gov/data-products/chart-gallery/gallery/chart-detail/?chartId=58388
[13] Available online at: www.fns.usda.gov/research-and-analysis.

eligibility requirements include four[14]. First, they must be in one of the targeted benefit categories: pregnant, postpartum, breastfeeding women, infants, or children under 5 years old. Second, they must have an official residence in the state where they apply for WIC benefits, and they must enroll at an authorized WIC clinic. Third, total household income must be less than or equal to 185% of the federal poverty income threshold. The income requirement could be satisfied through participation in certain programs, such as SNAP, Medicaid, or Temporary Assistance for Needy Families (TANF) programs. Lastly, applicants for the program must also have a diagnosed nutrition risk. WIC applicants who meet the four requirements are eligible for WIC benefits for six months and could extend their benefits for another six-month period. For children applicants, they will not be eligible after they arrive 5 years old. As for women applicants, they could be eligible during the nine months of pregnancy, and six months post-partum; for breastfeeding women, they could be eligible for up to one year after delivery.

Over the past decade, the WIC coverage rate, which refers to the percentage of eligible people who receive benefits, has generally declined, from 63.5% in 2011 to 51.1% in 2017, and this is true for all WIC target groups: infant, children, and women (USDA, 2020b). A report by the California Department of Public Health Multiple provides multiple reasons why eligible individuals do not enroll in WIC. The leading reason for pregnant women is that they do not think they qualify (40%), and the second leading reason is they do not think they need WIC (35%). Less common reasons include:

---

[14] USDA WIC Eligibility Requirements, URL: https://www.fns.usda.gov/wic/wic-eligibility-requirements

they do not know about WIC (16%), they have difficulty going to WIC clinics(14%), they have barriers to the application or telephone(10%), and they have a negative insight of WIC (9%) (California DPH, 2016). Jacknowitz and Tiehen (2007) show that participants who drop out of WIC early claim that taking part in WIC requires too much effort (25.7%), and they have problems with scheduling or transportation (10%). The language spoken by WIC staff is also found to be a participation barrier (Tiehen and Jacknowitz, 2008).

Several reasons are identified to explain the decline of WIC participation in recent years in the literature. First, improving economic conditions reduced the demand for WIC (Oliveira, 2017). Since WIC applicants need to earn an income equals to or below 185% of the poverty line or receive other assistance programs, the decrease of the unemployment rate and population in poverty may explain the drop. Second, the number of new birth dropped also reduces the potential WIC participants (Oliveira, 2017). Besides, there are also concerns among immigrant communities. In a fact sheet released by the New York State Department of Health, from 2009 to 2019, WIC enrollment decreased more steeply in neighborhoods with more non-citizen[15]. In this study, I also consider the county's economic condition and investigate whether the decrease of participation rate results from a better economy. I found that even considering economic condition, the decrease of WIC enrollment in Ohio is steeper than the decrease of population in poverty and unemployment.

---

[15] Retrieved from "Fact Sheet: WIC Enrollment Trends in New York City February 2020" https://www1.nyc.gov/assets/immigrants/downloads/pdf/fact-sheet-wic-enrollment-trends-february-2020.pdf

There are 16 food categories in the WIC food packages, which include "breakfast cereal, infant cereal, infant food fruits & vegetables, infant food meat, infant formula, exempt infant formula, milk, cheese, tofu, soy-based beverage, mature legumes, peanut butter, fruits & vegetables, canned fish, whole wheat bread and other whole grains, juice, eggs, WIC-eligible nutritionals and yogurt".[16] Notably, food packages are reevaluated every 10 years by the USDA.[17]

For fruits and vegetables, recipients are provided a certain amount of cash value through paper vouchers or EBT to only purchase fruits and vegetables in eligible grocery stores. All states were required to transit from paper voucher to EBT for WIC before October 2020. For the rest of the food categories, such as milk, juice, infant formula, WIC provides a certain amount of supplemental foods to recipients. The amount of each commodity differs by participant category.

Case studies show that WIC recipients do not make full use of their benefits. It is estimated that, from January to March 2012, on average, only 12.6% of WIC households used all of their food benefits in Kentucky, Michigan, and Nevada; the lowest rate is 9.5% in Kentucky. The highest one is 16.4% in Nevada (Phillips et al., 2014). Besides, about 5.3% of WIC households in these three states did not redeem their food benefits at all and ranged from 4.1% in Michigan to 8.0% in Nevada (Phillips et al., 2014).

[16] The WIC food packages are referenced from USDA: https://www.fns.usda.gov/wic/wic-food-packages-regulatory-requirements-wic-eligible-foods#FRUITS%20and%20VEGETABLES
[17] Retrieved from: https://www.nationalacademies.org/news/2017/01/revisions-to-wic-program-needed-changes-would-save-money-over-time

WIC redemption rates also vary across WIC participant categories and racial/ethnic and food categories. In Kentucky, Michigan, and Nevada, more than 25% of Asian households redeemed 100% of their WIC food in 2012, while only 8.9% of African American households made full use of their food (Phillips et al., 2014). The highest redemption rates in food categories include infant formula, milk, cash value benefit (CVB) for fruit and vegetables, and eggs. The lowest redemption rates in food categories are jarred baby meats, beans/peanut butter, infant cereal and jarred fruits and vegetables, and whole grains (Phillips et al., 2014).

Researchers have identified some of the barriers to WIC foods' redemption, such as negative interactions in stores, confusion over WIC rules, availability of products in allowable form, and feeling of embarrassment. For negative interactions in stores, researchers identified annoyance expressed by cashiers (Christie et al., 2006), cashiers' lack of training, and long waiting time (Bertmann et al., 2014; Gleason et al., 2014). As for confusion over WIC rules, gaps in knowledge (Bertmann et al., 2014; Gleason et al., 2014) is identified. It is also confirmed that availability of products in allowable form could be a barrier to benefit redemption, such as the limited selection of some WIC foods (Gleason et al., 2011), food package policies (Gleason et al., 2011), participants do not like the food or do not know how to cook them (Phillips et al., 2014). Lastly, feeling of embarrassment (Bertmann et al., 2014; Gleason et al., 2014) could also stop recipients from redeeming their benefit.

Given the overall decrease of enrollment and redemption of WIC in the U.S. This chapter aims to investigate the enrollment and redemption of WIC in Ohio at the county and participant category level and provide some insight into how and why the enrollment and redemption rate decrease. In this study, I use the administrative data from the Ohio Department of Health, Ohio Women Infants and Children Program (ODH) to identify the factors that correlate with participation and benefit redemption in the Ohio WIC program. As a result, I find a significant decrease in enrollment and redemption rate in Ohio from 2016 to 2018 at the county level.

3.2 Data

I use the administrative data from ODH to investigate the enrollment and redemption in WIC from March 2015 to February 2019. The data from ODH was pulled out from the database system, which compromised from multiple datasets: datasets that include participant information: participants, participants benefits, EBT card, EBT card balance, EBT clinic transaction, participant group, participant visit, clinic, and several datasets that explains about the variables encoding: annual income proof, breastfeeding ceased reason, breastfeeding frequency, certification status, change in smoking EBT message reason code, employment status, food category, food subcategory, health care source, income frequency, language, migrant status, participant category, participant transfer flag, pregnancy outcome, public assistance, racial-ethnic, referral, risk code, termination reason, and vitamin minerals. The participants were pulled out from the database system based on their certification dates, and these dates ranged from March 2nd, 2015 to February 28th, 2019. After obtaining the participants' unique id, their participant group, benefits, and EBT card balance were identified and pulled out from the database. In the participants data, demographic, geographic, and socio-economic information are included for each WIC participant, and their information is updated as their last visit. A detailed list of datasets and the variables in each dataset are provided in Appendix Table 45.

Notably, the administrative data I analyze do not have all WIC participants in Ohio for several reasons. First, to preserve privacy, ODH did not provide information on WIC participants residing in zip codes with fewer than 5 WIC participants. Second, due to ODH database record retention policies, some participant records get purged based on the date when ODH staff pull the data. Specifically, ODH policies require that the agency hold participant data for four years. Consequently, when ODH staff pull data based on a specific certification date, then records with dates as early as March 2015 get purged from the data. Third, due to WIC's recertification characteristics, some of the continuously enrolled participants – those who recertify on time – who had a recertification date after 2/28/2019 at the time ODH pulled their data are not included in my data set. This is because the WIC database system overwrites certification dates each time a participant recertifies instead of retaining all historical records. As a result, the data summary showed here is a subset of overall WIC participants in Ohio from March 2015 to February 2019.

3.3 Empirical Methodology

My main outcomes include enrollment and redemption rate in Ohio. In this section, I explain the methodologies I used to calculate enrollment and redemption.

Besides, the resources of covariates, such as population, the population in poverty, the population of unemployment by county, are also introduced.

I use the Participant Benefits table to calculate enrollment, which includes issued date, participant id, benefit year, benefit month, food category, food subcategory, effective date, quantity, and last update. I exclude individuals who have a zero entry for all benefit categories (521,052 cases), which means that though in the Participant Benefit dataset, they were assigned benefits in a certain month, but all the food category quantities are zero or less than zero. Thus, in fact, they did not receive any food benefits that month. Then, I calculate the number of unique participant ids for each benefit year and benefit month from March 2015 to Feb 2019 by month. For participant category (infant, child, pregnant woman, breastfeeding woman and not breastfeeding woman), because in the participant table, I only have participants' last updated category, I use their birth date, delivery date, and the time of receiving benefits to determine the real participant category at each month. For example, a child is categorized as a child in the participant dataset. In February 2019, when he is 2 years old, he is categorized as a child. He also received benefits in January 2018, at that month, he is categorized as an infant. A similar idea is used to change the participant category for breastfeeding women and not breastfeeding women; when receiving benefits is at least 10 months before the delivery time, the woman is identified as pregnant at that month.

I also consider the population in Ohio and the county's economic condition to investigate the WIC enrollment. I calculate the WIC participation rate using the number of participants per month divided by Ohio's population. I also calculate the participation rate by county by month with the county population. The population by county per year is retrieved from the United States Census Bureau[18]. Since I want to investigate whether the WIC enrollment rate is related to the economic condition, I also include county level unemployment rate and percent of the population below the poverty line in the analysis[19]. I calculate the ratio of WIC participants divided by the poverty population and the ratio of WIC participants divided by the unemployment population to check whether these two ratios increase or decrease in recent years, to show the relationship between participation and economic condition by county. For the county-level participation rate, since I have rates for each county per month for four consecutive years, I also use a county-level fixed effect model to investigate the rate trend.

The redemption rate is easy to calculate by food category based on the EBT card balance dataset. Each month, each EBT card, and each food category, there are issued quantity and available quantity. Issued quantity refers to in a certain month, for a certain food category, the participants who use this EBT card are assigned a certain amount. And available quantity refers to after redemption, how much is left unredeemed. However, it is hard to calculate the individual's redemption rate because WIC participants receive their food benefits through EBT as a participant group. There are at least one at most six participants in each participant group, and they receive their benefits with the same EBT card or two EBT cards. Thus, it is hard to estimate individual redemption condition since some participants share the EBT card balance.

---

[18] Retrieved from United States Census Bureau: https://www.census.gov/quickfacts/OH

[19] Retrieved from Ohio Department of Job and Family Services: https://ohiolmi.com/Home/RateMapArchive

3.4 Summary Statistics

In this section, I include several summary statistics that I conducted before the data visualization and regression.

First, a summary of percent of participant category by month is showed in Table 12. The overall average percent of child is about 48.8%, and infant is about 25.10%. For breastfeeding woman, not breastfeeding woman and pregnant woman, the percentage of participants are respectively 4.34%, 11.58% and 10.18%. The distribution is similar to the overall distribution of U.S. [20]

Table 12. Percentage of Participant Category by Month

	Woman Breastfeeding	Child (1-4)	Infant (0-1)	Woman not-Breastfeeding	Pregnant Woman
Mar-15	2.23%	54.23%	29.94%	3.77%	9.83%
Apr-15	2.25%	53.36%	29.46%	4.02%	10.90%
May-15	2.43%	51.19%	29.21%	4.38%	12.79%
Jun-15	2.94%	50.69%	28.31%	6.25%	11.82%
Jul-15	3.24%	51.00%	27.29%	7.28%	11.19%
Aug-15	3.47%	51.11%	26.38%	8.56%	10.48%
Sep-15	3.76%	51.44%	25.29%	9.86%	9.65%
Oct-15	3.89%	51.68%	24.59%	10.77%	9.07%
Nov-15	4.05%	51.94%	23.83%	11.63%	8.55%
Dec-15	4.05%	51.64%	24.15%	11.70%	8.47%
Jan-16	4.05%	51.43%	24.19%	11.81%	8.51%
Feb-16	4.10%	51.29%	24.29%	11.69%	8.64%
Mar-16	4.10%	50.88%	24.48%	11.57%	8.96%
Apr-16	4.10%	50.74%	24.44%	11.58%	9.13%
May-16	4.13%	50.61%	24.49%	11.55%	9.21%
Jun-16	4.13%	50.49%	24.48%	11.49%	9.41%
Jul-16	4.17%	50.21%	24.68%	11.46%	9.48%
Aug-16	4.18%	50.20%	24.63%	11.39%	9.60%

Continued

[20] The overall percentage of each participants category is retrieved from USDA: https://www.fns.usda.gov/wic/participant-and-program-characteristics-2018-charts

Continued Table 12

Sep-16	4.24%	50.28%	24.46%	11.57%	9.45%
Oct-16	4.27%	50.13%	24.54%	11.64%	9.43%
Nov-16	4.28%	50.00%	24.58%	11.75%	9.39%
Dec-16	4.30%	49.71%	24.86%	11.81%	9.32%
Jan-17	4.24%	49.30%	24.97%	11.89%	9.60%
Feb-17	4.25%	49.28%	24.95%	11.83%	9.68%
Mar-17	4.29%	48.98%	24.92%	11.57%	10.23%
Apr-17	4.30%	49.00%	24.78%	11.65%	10.27%
May-17	4.29%	48.66%	24.83%	11.47%	10.74%
Jun-17	4.32%	48.45%	24.76%	11.44%	11.03%
Jul-17	4.33%	48.24%	24.95%	11.35%	11.14%
Aug-17	4.31%	48.06%	25.03%	11.28%	11.32%
Sep-17	4.36%	48.06%	24.71%	11.66%	11.22%
Oct-17	4.47%	47.70%	24.77%	11.79%	11.27%
Nov-17	4.57%	47.41%	24.78%	12.16%	11.08%
Dec-17	4.71%	47.02%	24.98%	12.30%	10.99%
Jan-18	4.74%	46.38%	25.38%	12.19%	11.31%
Feb-18	4.77%	46.20%	25.65%	12.18%	11.20%
Mar-18	4.79%	46.01%	25.42%	12.17%	11.61%
Apr-18	4.96%	45.88%	25.14%	12.34%	11.69%
May-18	5.05%	45.46%	25.07%	12.41%	12.01%
Jun-18	5.17%	45.42%	24.63%	12.85%	11.93%
Jul-18	5.22%	45.11%	25.06%	12.97%	11.65%
Aug-18	5.33%	45.24%	25.24%	13.16%	11.03%
Sep-18	5.52%	45.80%	24.27%	14.21%	10.20%
Oct-18	5.47%	45.96%	23.60%	15.07%	9.91%
Nov-18	5.51%	45.77%	23.07%	16.42%	9.22%
Dec-18	5.59%	45.13%	22.95%	17.39%	8.65%
Jan-19	5.68%	44.89%	23.82%	17.45%	8.15%
Feb-19	5.83%	44.61%	24.47%	17.08%	8.01%
Average	4.34%	48.80%	25.10%	11.58%	10.18%

Then in Table 13, I show the average redemption rate by participant category. In this table, I only include the participants who do not share EBT card with others, because I can only identify individual redemption rate for those participants. Overall, I find that breastfeeding woman category has the highest average redemption rate as about 64.80%, while pregnant woman category has the lowest average redemption rate as about 58.87%.

Table 13. The Average Redemption Rate for Each Participant Category

Participant Category	Average Redemption Rate	Std.dev.
Woman Breastfeeding	64.80%	0.44
Child (1-4)	63.03%	0.44
Infant (0-1)	64.10%	0.45
Woman not-Breastfeeding	61.34%	0.45
Pregnant Woman	58.87%	0.45

In Table 14, I show the average redemption rate for all food categories and all participants by month, and overall, it shows a decrease trend of redemption from 2015 to 2019.

Table 14. Average Redemption Rate by Month

Year/Month	Average Redemption Rate	[95% Conf.Interval]	
201505	65.14%	64.83%	65.45%
201506	69.47%	69.24%	69.69%
201507	68.44%	68.27%	68.61%
201508	69.15%	69.01%	69.29%
201509	66.90%	66.77%	67.02%
201510	66.01%	65.89%	66.13%
201511	65.55%	65.43%	65.67%
201512	64.99%	64.87%	65.11%
201601	67.66%	67.54%	67.78%
201602	63.51%	63.39%	63.63%
201603	63.99%	63.87%	64.11%
201604	63.36%	63.24%	63.49%
201605	64.79%	64.66%	64.91%
201606	64.16%	64.04%	64.28%
201607	65.03%	64.91%	65.16%
201608	65.17%	65.05%	65.30%

Continued

Continued Table 14

201609	63.09%	62.96%	63.21%
201610	63.39%	63.27%	63.52%
201611	62.79%	62.66%	62.91%
201612	62.48%	62.35%	62.60%
201701	65.00%	64.87%	65.12%
201702	61.38%	61.26%	61.51%
201703	61.21%	61.08%	61.33%
201704	61.03%	60.90%	61.16%
201705	62.60%	62.47%	62.73%
201706	61.14%	61.01%	61.27%
201707	62.87%	62.74%	63.00%
201708	62.98%	62.85%	63.11%
201709	60.14%	60.01%	60.27%
201710	61.92%	61.79%	62.05%
201711	60.95%	60.82%	61.08%
201712	60.36%	60.22%	60.49%
201801	63.47%	63.34%	63.61%
201802	59.16%	59.03%	59.30%
201803	58.91%	58.78%	59.05%
201804	59.39%	59.25%	59.53%
201805	59.62%	59.48%	59.75%
201806	58.59%	58.45%	58.72%
201807	60.69%	60.55%	60.82%
201808	59.34%	59.20%	59.48%
201809	58.21%	58.07%	58.35%
201810	58.19%	58.05%	58.33%
201811	56.30%	56.16%	56.45%
201812	56.48%	56.33%	56.63%
201901	57.13%	56.98%	57.28%
201902	54.89%	54.74%	55.05%
Average	62.33%		

3.5 Results

3.5.1 WIC Enrollment in Ohio

I use WIC benefits to estimate the number of monthly WIC participants in Ohio from August 2015 to February 2019, then I divide this number of participants by the state population and multiply by 10,000 to estimate the participation rate in Ohio per 10,000 population. I also conduct similar calculations on the county level. Overall, I find a decreasing trend of WIC enrollment in Ohio and in almost every county in Ohio, which is similar to the WIC enrollment in the U.S as a whole[21]. To show the trend, I do not only visualize the enrollment in the state and county level but also conduct fixed effect regression to confirm. Apart from enrollment by county, I also analyze WIC enrollment by participant category and racial/ethnic.

Figure 1 shows the trend of the number of WIC participants in Ohio by month, and Figure 2 shows the trend of WIC participants per 10,000 people in Ohio by month. Figure 1 also showed the official number of WIC participants published by USDA and verified by ODH[22]. I explained the discrepancy between the two series in the previous section, and the main reason for the spike in numbers in 2015 results from the purging that explained in the previous section. Overall, I find a decreasing trend in the number of monthly participants and the number of participants per 10,000 Ohio residents since November 2015. On average, the participation rate per 10,000 Ohio residents is about

[21] National Level Monthly Data retrieved from USDA: https://fns-prod.azureedge.net/sites/default/files/resource-files/37WIC_Monthly-7.pdf

[22] Ohio Monthly Data – State Level Participation by Category retrieved from: https://www.fns.usda.gov/pd/wic-program

15.2. The highest participation rate per 10,000 Ohio residents in this time period is about 19.2 in November 2015, and the lowest participation rate is about 9.3 in February 2019.

Figure 8. Enrollment of WIC in Ohio

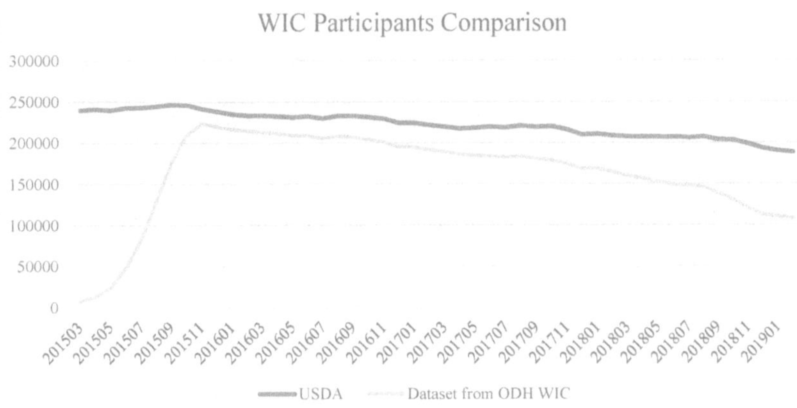

Figure 9. Number of participants/1,000 residents in Ohio

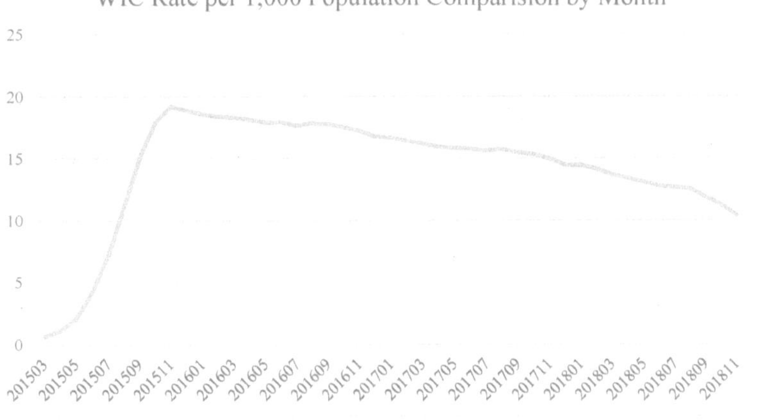

Ohio includes a diverse set of counties ranging from densely populated urban centers such as Columbus and Cleveland to more sparsely populated areas, such as Athens. Besides, the south-eastern counties along the Kentucky/West Virginia/Pennsylvania borders make up part of rural Appalachia. This area has its own set of challenges, including opioid misuse and high unemployment (Betz and Jones, 2018). WIC eligible women and children could greatly benefit from the program.

To investigate variation in participation across counties and make sure declines in the population do not drive declines in WIC participation. I calculate county-level participation per 10,000 with county participant totals divided by county population[23]. Figure 10 is a heat map of the WIC participation per 10,000 county residents. Shades of darker blue represent higher participation per 10,000 county residents, and lighter blue shades represent the opposite. I also plot these heat maps from 2015 through 2019. Overall, I find a decreasing trend of participation per 10,000 county residents among all counties. There does not seem to be a single county or set of counties driving the decrease in participation. For each year, I annotate counties with the highest and lowest participation per 10,000 county residents. Vinton has the highest participation from 2015-2019, and Delaware has the lowest participation. I also find higher participation per 10,000 county residents in the south area of Ohio, which includes Vinton, Highland, Pike, Lawrence, and Scioto.

[23] Notes: I only use county level population by year, for the number of participants, I have it by month.

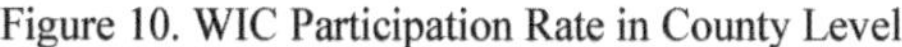

Figure 10. WIC Participation Rate in County Level

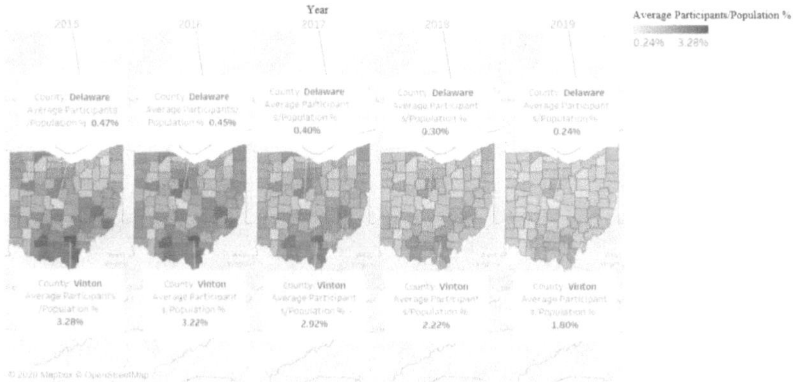

To show the change of participation rate by year, I calculate the percent change of participation rate by dividing the participation rate for this year by last year and then minus 1. In Figure 11, I demonstrate these changes with heat maps across years. In these maps, shades of blue represent an increase in participation rate compared to the last year, and shades of orange represent declines in participation rate. The map for 2015 is grey because I do not have data for 2014. In 2016, I find almost half of the counties in Ohio have higher participation rate than in 2015, and the highest rate is Summit County, which increases about 46.47%. Summit County is an urban county with the fourth-most populous county in Ohio in the Census 2010, and compared with other counties, its population below poverty line and unemployment population is not extreme high or low. From 2017-2019, I find all counties with decreases of participation rate. For each year, I annotate counties with highest and lowest percent changes.

Figure 11. Percent Change of WIC Participation Rate in County Level

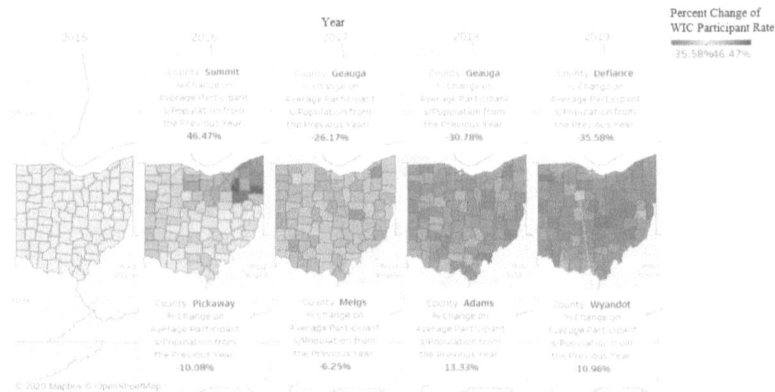

It is possible that the decreasing trend of participation rate in Ohio is related to an improved economy. As incomes increase, people may no longer need WIC benefits. As a way to test the validity of this hypothesis I use several indicators of economic strength including the unemployment rate and the percent of the population (state and county) at or below the poverty threshold. In Figure 12, I plot several series to illustrate the relationship between economic indicators and WIC participation. To visualize these relationships, I calculate the ratio of WIC participants to total population and divide that ratio by the unemployment rate or the percent of population under the poverty threshold.

In Figure 12, I show a slightly decreasing trend for the percent of the population below the poverty level and a slightly decreasing unemployment rate from 2016 to 2018. As another economic indicator, I also plot per capita income from 2015 to 2019 (not adjusted). Notably, however, I observe a steeper declines in WIC participants per unemployed and WIC participants per individuals in poverty than in the indicators themselves. This seems to suggest that a stronger economy only captures a portion of the variation in WIC enrollment.

Figure 12. The Trends of WIC Participation with Economic Condition in Ohio by Year

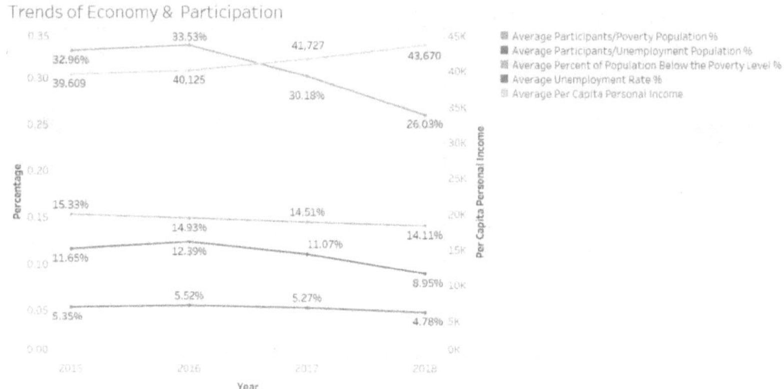

To investigate county-level WIC participation per unemployed individual how these ratios change over time. I include these outcomes in Figure 13. In this heat map, darker shades of blue represent higher ratios of participation divided by unemployment population, which means that more people in need are enrolled in WIC in this county. I annotate counties with highest and lowest ratios for each year.

Figure 13. WIC Participation with Unemployment Population in Ohio by Year by County

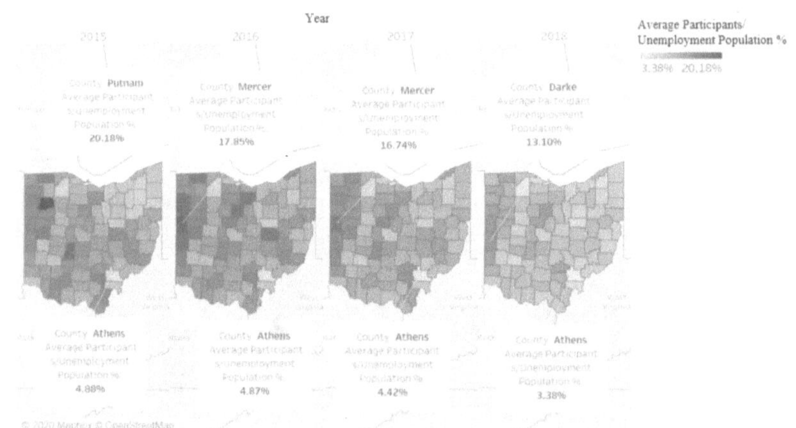

To investigate the participation rate by county, I have a heat map in Figure 14 showing the ratio of participation and poverty population by county by year. Here, darker blue refers higher ratio of participation divided by population below poverty line, which means that more people in need are enrolled in WIC in this county. I annotate counties with highest and lowest ratios for each year.

Figure 14. WIC Participation with Population in Poverty in Ohio by Year by County

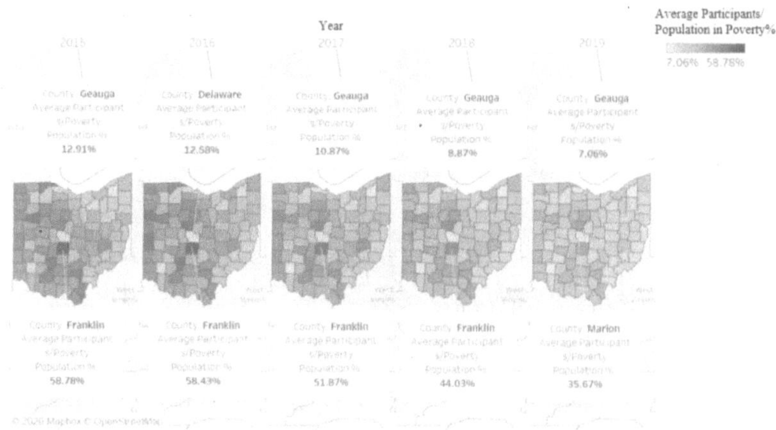

In Figure 15, I show the WIC participants components by month from August 2015 to February 2019. Generally, there are almost half of WIC participants are children, and 25% of infants. A decreasing trend of participation is also shown in this chart.

Figure 15. WIC Participation Shares over Time

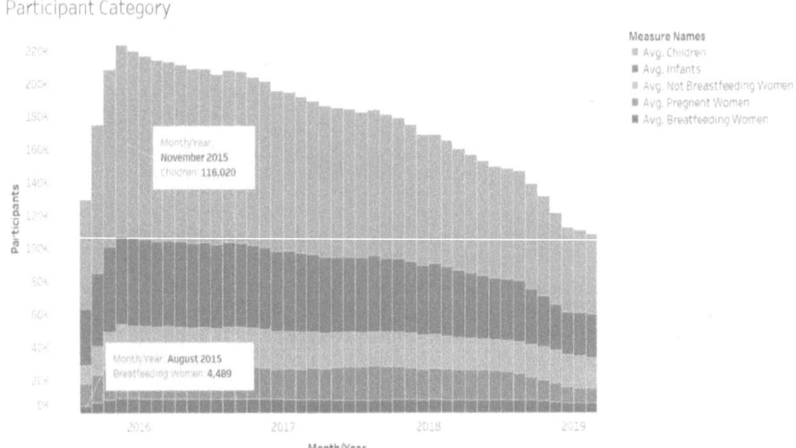

2019. Generally, there are almost half of WIC participants are children, and 25% of infants. A decreasing trend of participation is also shown in this chart.

In Figure 16, I show the number of WIC participants by racial/ethnic by month from August 2015 to February 2019. There is a decreasing trend among all the subgroups, which also shows that the decreasing of WIC enrollment does not result from the decreasing of any one subgroup of racial/ethnic.

Figure 16. WIC Participation by Racial/Ethnic in Ohio

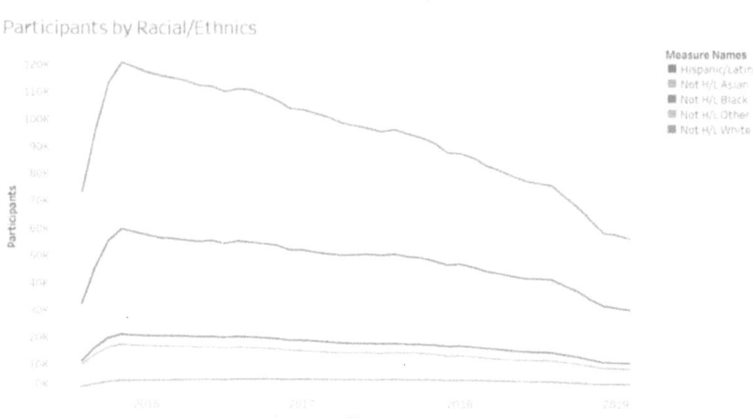

Based on the comparison between USDA data and the data I have from Ohio ODH, I find that I have more similar number of participants and decrease trend from November 2015 to December 2017. Thus, I use monthly WIC enrollment during this time period to conduct regression data analysis.

I firstly regress the monthly WIC participation rate in the Ohio (from November 2015 to December 2017) on year fixed effect and month as time trend for data from USDA and ODH. Table 15 shows that, compared with 2015, WIC participation rate (number of WIC participant divided by population) decreased significantly in 2016 and 2017, in both two data sources.

Table 15. Relationship between WIC Enrollment Rate in Ohio and Time

VARIABLES	(1) WIC Enrollment Rate (USDA)	(2) WIC Enrollment Rate (ODH)
2016. Year	-0.00104***	-0.00225***
	(0.000142)	(0.000316)
2017. Year	-0.00218***	-0.00441***
	(0.000142)	(0.000316)
month	-5.97e-05***	-0.000207***
	(8.86e-06)	(1.98e-05)
Observations	26	26
Year fixed effect	YES	YES
Month Time Trend	YES	YES

Standard errors in parentheses: *** $p<0.01$, ** $p<0.05$, * $p<0.1$

For WIC enrollment in the county level, I also conduct fixed effect regression to show the decrease trend. In Table16, I regress number of participants by county (column 1) and number of participants per 1,000 population by county (column 2) on year fixed effect and month as time trend.

Table 16. Relationship between Number of WIC Participants, Enrollment Rate by County and Time in Ohio

VARIABLES	(1) # of participants by county	(2) participants/1000population by county
2016.Year	-255.4***	-2.170***
	(25.74)	(0.0634)
2017.Year	-535.8***	-4.590***
	(25.74)	(0.0634)
Month	-19.66***	-0.182***
	(1.857)	(0.00457)
Observations	2,288	2,288
Number of county	88	88
County fixed effect	YES	YES
Year fixed effect	YES	YES
Month time trend	YES	YES

Standard errors in parentheses: *** p<0.01, ** p<0.05, * p<0.1

Taking economic condition into consideration, I create one ratio as participation population divided by poverty population, another ratio as participation population divided by unemployment population in county level to check whether people drop WIC because they do not need WIC benefits any more. I also conduct fixed effect regression on these two ratios, and find that compared with 2015, both ratios decreased significantly in 2016 and 2017, showing that less ratio of people in poverty got enrolled in WIC, and less people in unemployment got enrolled in WIC. And also confirm that the reason that less people get enrolled in WIC is not result from better economic condition.

Table 17. Relationship between Number of WIC Participants, Enrollment Rate by County and Time in Ohio

VARIABLES	(1) participants/unemployment by county	(2) participants/poverty population by county
2016.Year	-0.0479***	-0.0119***
	(0.00141)	(0.000536)
2017.Year	-0.0818***	-0.0254***
	(0.00141)	(0.000536)
Month	-0.00341***	-0.00127***
	(0.000102)	(3.87e-05)
Observations	2,288	2,288
R-squared	0.690	0.659
Number of counties	88	88
County fixed effect	YES	YES
Year fixed effect	YES	YES
Month time trend	YES	YES

Standard errors in parentheses: *** p<0.01, ** p<0.05, * p<0.1

3.3.2 Redemption Rate of WIC Benefits

I investigate about redemption of WIC participants over time in Figure 10. Breastfeeding women have the highest redemption rate, while pregnant women have the lowest. Overall, there is a decrease trend of redemption in all categories of WIC participants.

Figure 17. The Redemption Rate by participant Group over Time

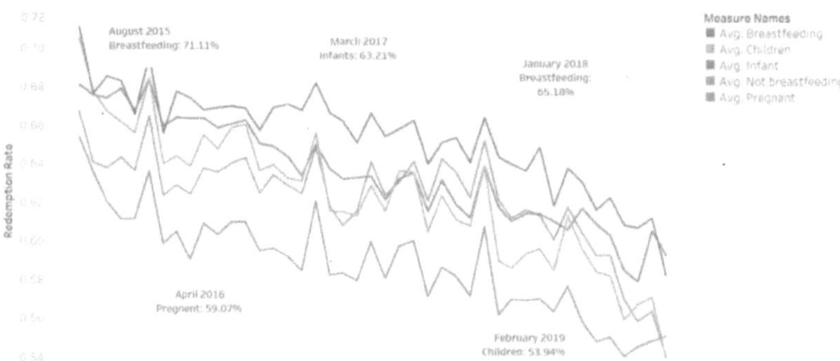

In Figure 18, 19 and 20, I show the redemption rate for all the food categories that in WIC packages. I find a pretty flat redemption rate for the infant formula, but decrease trends of redemption rate for the rest of food categories.

Figure 18. Redemption Rate by Food Category over Time (a)

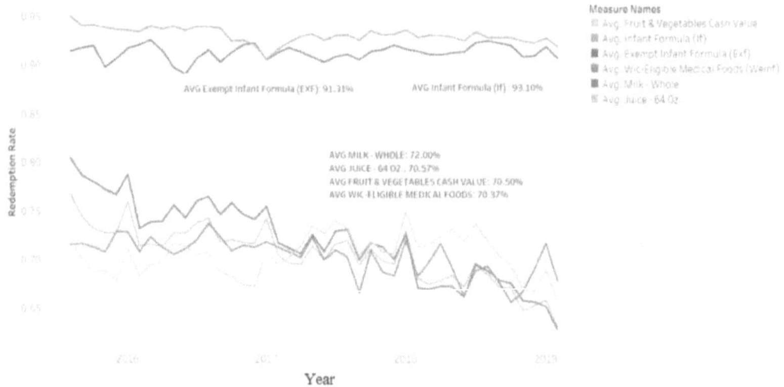

Figure 19. Redemption Rate by Food Category over Time (b)

Measure Names
Avg. Cheese Or Tofu
Avg. Eggs
Avg. Breakfast Cereal
Avg. Infant Fruits & Veg 4 Oz
Avg. Milk 1%, 1/2%, Skim
Avg. Frozen Juice 11.5 Oz. Or 12 Oz.
AVG EGGS: 69.97%
AVG MILK 1%, 1/2%, SKIM: 62.44%
AVG CHEESE OR TOFU: 61.49%
AVG INFANT FRUITS & VEG 4 OZ.: 58.52%
AVG FROZEN JUICE 11.5 OZ. OR 12 OZ.: 57.05%
AVG BREAKFAST CEREAL: 54.61%
Redemption Rate
Year

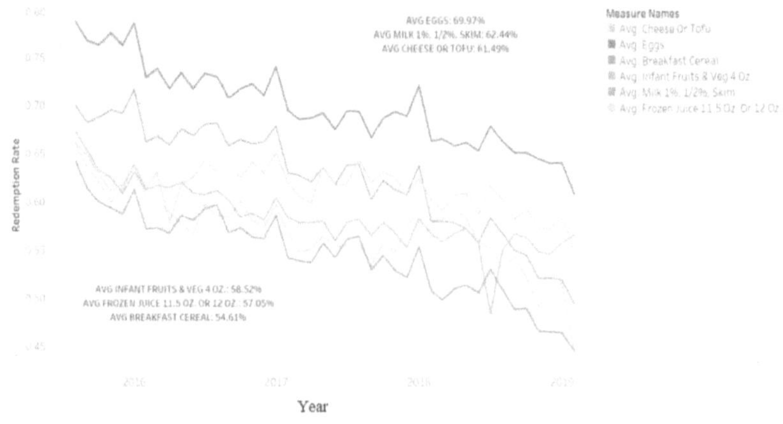

Figure 20. Redemption Rate by Food Category over Time (c)

Measure Names
Legumes
Fish
Infant Cereal
Infant Meats 2.5 Oz.
Bread/Whole Grains
AVG FISH: 53.99%
AVG INFANT CEREAL: 49.89%
AVG LEGUMES: 48.95%
AVG BREAD/WHOLE GRAINS: 49.35%
AVG INFANT MEATS
2.5 OZ.: 34.36%
Redemption Rate
Year

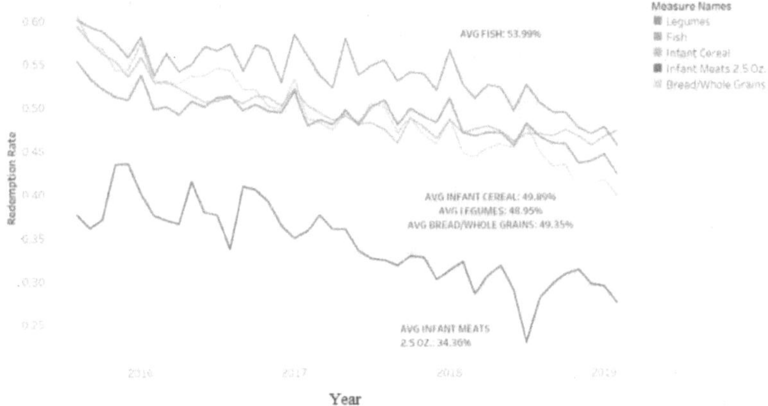

In the Figure 21, I show the average redemption rate in Ohio by racial/ethnic group, and I find that overall Asian participants redeem the most of their benefits, and not Hispanic/Latino African American redeem the least.

Figure 21. The Average Redemption Rate by Racial/Ethnic Group

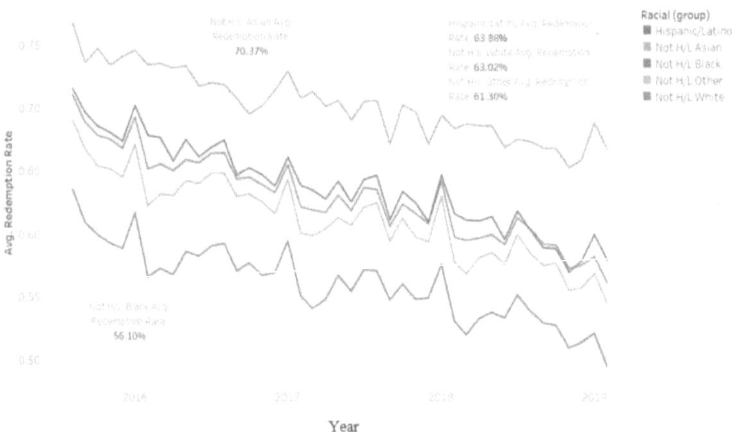

For redemption rate in the county level, I also conduct fixed-effect model to investigate about the decreasing trend. In Table 18, I regress average monthly redemption rate by county on year fixed effect and month as time trend. Overall, I find compared with 2016, the average redemption rate in 2017 and 2018 are statistically significant lower in county level.

Table 18. Relationship between Average Monthly Redemption Rate by County and Time in Ohio

VARIABLES	(1) Redemption Rate
2017.Year	-0.0292***
	(0.00122)
2018.Year	-0.0499***
	(0.00147)
Month	-0.00221***
	(9.40e-05)
Observations	3,168
Number of counties	88
Adjusted R-squared	0.578
County fixed effect	YES
Year fixed effect	YES
Month time trend	YES

Robust standard errors in parentheses: *** p<0.01, ** p<0.05, * p<0.1

I also conduct similar fixed effect regression on county level redemption rate for all the food categories to check whether the redemption rate of some food categories does not decrease as others. I analyze all the food categories in the dataset: eggs, breakfast cereal, legumes, fish, bread/whole grains, and WIC-eligible medical foods in Table 19, cheese or tofu, milk-whole, Milk-1%, 1/2%, skim, fruits &vegetables cash value, juice and frozen juice in Table 20, infant cereal, infant fruits &vegetables, infant meats, infant formula, exempt infant formula in Table 21. I find that the average redemption rate of cash value fruits and vegetables increased significantly in 2017 and 2018, compared to 2016 in the county level. And the average redemption rate of exempt infant formula increased significantly in 2018 compared to 2016. For the rest of food categories, they all decreased statistically significant in 2017 and 2018, compared to 2016 in the county level.

Table 19. Relationship between Average Monthly Redemption Rate by County and Time in Ohio (a)

VARIABLES	(1) Eggs	(2) Breakfast Cereal	(3) Legumes	(4) Fish	(5) Bread/Whole Grains	(6) WIC-Eligible Medical Foods
2017.Year	-0.0421***	-0.0404***	-0.0199***	-0.0314***	-0.0495***	-0.0287***
	(0.00118)	(0.00108)	(0.00112)	(0.00389)	(0.00124)	(0.00538)
2018.Year	-0.0611***	-0.0748***	-0.0386***	-0.0589***	-0.0863***	-0.0328***
	(0.00125)	(0.00112)	(0.00114)	(0.00406)	(0.00132)	(0.00570)
Month	-0.00255***	-0.00251***	-0.00136***	-0.00352***	-0.00362***	-0.00238***
	(0.000162)	(0.000136)	(0.000146)	(0.000476)	(0.000152)	(0.000669)
Adjusted R-squared	0.634	0.748	0.722	0.206	0.740	0.200
Number of Counties	88	88	88	88	88	88
County fixed effect	YES	YES	YES	YES	YES	YES
Year fixed effect	YES	YES	YES	YES	YES	YES
Month time trend	YES	YES	YES	YES	YES	YES

Robust standard errors in parentheses: *** $p<0.01$, ** $p<0.05$, * $p<0.1$

Table 20. Relationship between Average Monthly Redemption Rate by County and Time in Ohio (b)

VARIABLES	(1) Cheese or Tofu	(2) Milk-Whole	(3) Milk-1%, 1/2%, Skim	(4) Fruits &Vegetables Cash Value	(5) Juice	(6) Frozen Juice
2017.Year	-0.0189***	-0.0367***	-0.0367***	0.00948***	-0.0259***	-0.0454***
	(0.00355)	(0.00149)	(0.00149)	(0.00111)	(0.00107)	(0.00742)
2018.Year	-0.0545***	-0.0656***	-0.0656***	0.0147***	-0.0489***	-0.0611***
	(0.00374)	(0.00159)	(0.00159)	(0.00108)	(0.00116)	(0.00756)
Month	-0.00197***	-0.00143***	-0.00143***	-0.00268***	-0.00188***	-0.00402***
	(0.000436)	(0.000197)	(0.000197)	(0.000133)	(0.000142)	(0.000921)
Adjusted R-squared	0.258	0.563	0.563	0.641	0.571	0.155
Number of Counties	88	88	88	88	88	88
County fixed effect	YES	YES	YES	YES	YES	YES
Year fixed effect	YES	YES	YES	YES	YES	YES
Month time trend	YES	YES	YES	YES	YES	YES

Robust standard errors in parentheses: *** p<0.01, ** p<0.05, * p<0.1

Table 21. Relationship between Average Monthly Redemption Rate by County and Time in Ohio (c)

VARIABLES	(1) Infant Cereal	(2) Infant Fruits &Vegetables	(3) Infant Meats	(4) Infant Formula	(5) Exempt Infant Formula
2017.Year	-0.0316***	-0.0277***	-0.0319***	-0.0119***	-1.91e-05
	(0.00208)	(0.00178)	(0.00616)	(0.000870)	(0.00229)
2018.Year	-0.0533***	-0.0474***	-0.0778***	-0.00999***	0.00450**
	(0.00210)	(0.00191)	(0.00668)	(0.000839)	(0.00225)
Month	-0.00285***	-0.00241***	-0.00102	-0.000198*	3.33e-05
	(0.000257)	(0.000218)	(0.000774)	(0.000108)	(0.000269)
Adjusted R-squared	0.441	0.474	0.126	0.162	0.081
Number of Counties	88	88	88	88	88
County fixed effect	YES	YES	YES	YES	YES
Year fixed effect	YES	YES	YES	YES	YES
Month time trend	YES	YES	YES	YES	YES

Robust standard errors in parentheses: *** $p<0.01$, ** $p<0.05$, * $p<0.1$

3.6 Conclusion and Limitations

In this Chapter, I investigate the enrollment and redemption of WIC in Ohio at county, and participant category level. With the administrative data from ODH WIC, population and economic data, I confirm a decrease trend of enrollment rate and redemption rate in Ohio from 2015 to 2018. The enrollment rate declined both in county and participant category level, so the decline does not result from the decline in several counties or single participant group. In addition, I also consider about the economic condition by county and find that the decrease of participation rate does not result from less population in poverty or unemployment. Apart from these, I analyze the enrollment and redemption by racial/ethnic, and confirm that the decrease of both enrollment and redemption rate do not result from the decrease in certain racial/ethnic group. To investigate the decrease trend of redemption rate, I analyzed county level redemption rate by food categories, and find a decrease trend for most food categories, except cash value fruits and vegetables, and exempt infant formula. One of the biggest limitation of this study is the problem of subsampling, in the future work, similar analysis and calculation could be used on new data from ODH.

Chapter 4. The Impact of the Duration of WIC Enrollment on Health Outcomes

4.1 Introduction

In 2017, 11.8% of US households experienced food insecurity during some time of the year[24]. Unfortunately, food insecurity can have detrimental effects on adults and children. For example, for children, food insecurity is found to cause physical health problems: general health (Gundersen & Kreider, 2009), congenital disabilities (Carmichael et al., 2007), non-cognitive problems (Howard, 2011), asthma (Kirkpatrick, 2010), oral health (Chi, et al., 2014); psychological problems: depression (Melchior, 2012), aggression, anxiety (Whitaker et a., 2006), suicide ideation (McIntyre, 2013), behavior problems (Huang et al., 2010); academic performance (Alaimo et al., 2001), social skills (Jyoti et al., 2005). As for adults, many studies show the association of food insecurity and nutrition intakes, physical health problems: general health condition (Vozoris & Tarasuk, 2003), bad health exams performance(Stuff et al., 2004), oral health problems (Muirhead et al., 2009), sleep problems (Ding et al., 2014), diabetes (Seligman et al., 2007).; psychological problems: mental health problems (Heflin et al., 2005), depression (Casey et al., 2004).

---

[24] The data source: https://www.ers.usda.gov/topics/food-nutrition-assistance/food-security-in-the-us/key-statistics-graphics.aspx#foodsecure

To reduce the negative effects of food insecurity, the federal government currently authorizes 15 different nutrition assistance programs, and in the fiscal year, 2019 spent $92.4 billion.[25] Among these programs, WIC falls third in terms of costs – behind the SNAP and School Lunch Program (NSLP)— and provides benefits to some of society's most vulnerable members.

In general, empirical evidence on the impact of WIC tends to fall into three categories: 1) whether or not WIC participation successfully reduces food insecurity; 2) whether, and to what extent, WIC influences consumption patterns; and 3) which health outcomes are most impacted by participation in WIC. Empirical evidence of the benefits of WIC show that WIC reduces food insecurity (Black et l., 2004; Kreider et al., 2016; Metallinos-Katsaras et al., 2011), affect participants' consumption pattern by increasing their consumption in fruit juice (Vercammen et al., 2018), cereal and grains (Oh, Jensen and Rahkovsky, 2016; Khan et al., 2018), and improve both birth (Hoynes, Page and Stevens, 2011; Currie and Rajani in 2015) and children outcomes (Chorniy, Currie and Sonchak, 2018; Jackson, 2015).

In this chapter, I intend to expand on previous work by exploring the effect of time length that children stay in WIC on their health outcomes: the number of risk conditions and BMI percentile. This study is important for several reasons. First, an eligible child could receive WIC benefits from birth (as an infant from 0 to 1) to age 5 (as a child from 1 to 5), which could be a great number of food benefits. While the program

[25] The data source: https://www.ers.usda.gov/data-products/chart-gallery/gallery/chart-detail/?chartId=58388

delivers benefits to about 84% of WIC-eligible infants, but only about 53% of WIC-eligible children. The results of this research could emphasize the effect of WIC on children's health outcomes and assistant with reducing eligible children drop-out. Second, WIC plays an essential role in improving the health of a large number of vulnerable populations. The results of this research could support and encourage WIC enrollment and program utilization.

In this study, I use the administrative data from the Ohio Department of Health (ODH) WIC, the same data used in Chapter 2, to investigate the impact of WIC length on children's health outcomes. In the data, most WIC participants in Ohio were assigned WIC benefits from March 2015 to February 2019. Due to some reasons, the data I have does not include all the Ohio participants, and the reasons are explained in the data part in Chapter 2. From the administrative data, I have participants' demographic information and their health condition every time they visit the clinic during the time they are in WIC. Compared with the datasets used in other WIC research, the administrative data includes detailed participants' information and their longitudinal, accurate health condition measured by the WIC clinic, which reduces the possibility of self-reported bias under-reporting of WIC participation.

I use the length of time that a child enrolled in WIC as a source of exogenous variation and determine if those on the program longer do better in health outcomes. Since I have panel data on each participant, I use a fixed-effect model to solve the unobservable variation that affects children's health. The health outcomes used in this research include the number of risk conditions and BMI percentile.

4.2 Overview of WIC

As the third-largest federal nutrition assistance program, WIC targets low-income women, infants, and children under age 5 who are at nutrition risk. In April 2018, 7.8 million people participated in WIC (Kline et al., 2020). Of these participants, 1.87 million were infants, 4.15 million were children under the age of 5, and 1.81 million were pregnant, breastfeeding, and postpartum women.[26] When considered in the context of the US population, WIC serves approximately 51% of all infants, 28.4% of all children under the age of five, and over one forth of all pregnant and postpartum women (Oliveira & Frazao, 2015). In 2019 these services cost the federal government nearly $5.2 billion, with about 39.8% directed to program overhead, and 60.2% directed to actual benefit receipts.[27]

WIC applicants must meet four main requirements to qualify for benefits.[28] First, they must be in one of the targeted benefit groups: pregnant, postpartum, breastfeeding women, infants, or children under 5 years old. Second, they must have an official residence in the state where they apply for WIC benefits, and they must enroll at an authorized WIC clinic. Third, total household income must be less than or equal to 185% of the federal poverty income threshold. However, the income requirement could also be satisfied through participation in certain programs, such as SNAP, Medicaid, or TANF programs. Lastly, WIC applicants for the program need to have a diagnosed nutrition

---

[26] Available online at: www.fns.usda.gov/research-and-analysis.

[27] The data is retrieved from USDA: https://fns-prod.azureedge.net/sites/default/files/resource-files/wisummary-7.pdf

[28] The general requirements are based on USDA, each state may has various process of application. https://www.fns.usda.gov/wic/wic-eligibility-requirements

risk. WIC clinicians determine these risks in the initial consultation. Nutrition risks are usually medical-based or dietary-based conditions. Guidelines from the National Academy of Medicine (NAM), previously named the Institute of Medicine (IOM), characterize nutrition risk into five broad categories: anthropometric (such as low weight-for-height), biochemical (such as low elevated blood lead level), clinical/health/medical (such as chronic, genetic diseases), dietary (such as inadequate nutrition intake), or other (such as homelessness).[29] Each of these general categories contains multiple subgroups WIC clinicians use to designate a specific nutrition risk.

The nutrition risk designation is an important mechanism for allocating limited WIC funding to benefit those most in need. Yet, in more recent years, clinicians have applied a more relaxed definition of nutrition risk, resulting in a larger pool of eligible individuals. For example, if an individual is underweight, or has a history of poor birth outcomes, or has a poor diet, this individual qualifies for WIC. Furthermore, empirical evidence shows that WIC clinicians record all applicants as meeting the nutrition risk requirement (Bitler, Currie, and Scholz, 2003). Once applicants meet all the requirements and begin receiving benefits, they must recertify on a 6-month or annual basis[30].

Authorized food benefits in the WIC program is different from those in the SNAP program. Each month, SNAP recipients receive a pre-determined amount of money they access through an Electronic Benefits Transfer (EBT) card. SNAP policy authorizes recipients to use the funds to purchase most food and beverage types, excluding alcoholic

---

[29] Institute of Medicine (US). Committee on Dietary Risk Assessment in the WIC Program. (2002), available at: https://fns-prod.azureedge.net/sites/default/files/WICDietaryRisk.pdf
[30] The regulation is retrieved from USDA WIC: https://www.fns.usda.gov/wic/who-gets-wic-and-how-apply

beverages, medicine, or pre-made foods[31]. Similar to the SNAP program, WIC recipients access benefits through vouchers or an EBT card. In contrast, however, WIC authorizes only a specific set of commodities recipients can redeem with benefits, and each commodity has quantity limits. Notably, while SNAP recipients receive a direct cash transfer with limitations on what the funds can purchase, WIC recipients receive a set quantity of specific commodities each month. For example, a WIC child under five years old can get one dozen eggs, 16 quarts of milk, and 36 ounces of cereals per month. Authorized WIC commodities fall into 16 different food categories: breakfast cereal, infant cereal, infant fruits & vegetables, infant meat, infant formula, exempt infant formula, milk, cheese, tofu, soy-based beverages, mature legumes, peanut butter, fruits & vegetables, canned fish, whole wheat bread and other whole grains, juice, eggs, WIC-eligible nutritionals, and yogurt.[32] I report the maximum monthly allowances of WIC food in Tables 1 and 2. For fruits and vegetables, each WIC recipients receive a certain amount of cash to purchase any eligible fresh or processed fruits and vegetables. Recipients receive this cash either via paper vouchers or EBT card benefits. Based on the federal Healthy, Hunger-Free Kids Act of 2010, all states must distribute WIC benefits using the EBT system instead of paper vouchers. And in Ohio, this transition was conducted from 2014 to 2015 in all the counties gradually.

[31] From what can SNAP buy: https://www.fns.usda.gov/snap/eligible-food-items

[32] The WIC food packages are referenced from USDA: https://www.fns.usda.gov/wic/wic-food-packages-regulatory-requirements-wic-eligible-foods#FRUITS%20and%20VEGETABLES

Table 22. WIC food Package (a)[33]

SNAPSHOT of the WIC Food Packages [1]				
Maximum Monthly Allowances of Supplemental Foods for Children and Women				
Foods	Children	Women		
	Food Package IV 1 through 4 years	Food Package V: Pregnant and Partially (Mostly) Breastfeeding (up to 1 year postpartum)	Food Package VI: Postpartum (up to 6 months postpartum)	Food Package VII: Fully Breastfeeding (up to 1 year post-partum)
Juice, single strength	128 fl oz	144 fl oz	96 fl oz	144 fl oz
Milk [2]	16 qt	22 qt	16 qt	24 qt
Breakfast cereal [3]	36 oz	36 oz	36 oz	36 oz
Cheese	N/A	N/A	N/A	1 lb
Eggs	1 dozen	1 dozen	1 dozen	2 dozen
Fruits and vegetables	$8.00 in cash value vouchers	$11.00 in cash value vouchers	$11.00 in cash value vouchers	$11.00 in cash value vouchers
Whole wheat bread [4]	2 lb	1 lb	N/A	1 lb
Fish (canned) [5]	N/A	N/A	N/A	30 oz
Legumes, dry or canned and/or Peanut butter	1 lb (64 oz canned) Or 18 oz	1 lb (64 ounce canned) And 18 oz	1 lb (64 ounce canned) Or 18 oz	1 lb (64 ounce canned) And 18 oz

[1] Refer to the full regulation at ***www.fns.usda.gov/wic*** for the complete provisions and requirements for WIC foods.
[2] Allowable options for fluid milk substitutions are yogurt, cheese, soy beverage, and tofu.
[3] At least one half of the total number of breakfast cereals on State agency food list must be whole grain.
[4] Allowable options for whole wheat bread are whole grain bread, brown rice, bulgur, oatmeal, whole-grain barley, whole wheat macaroni products, or soft corn or whole wheat tortillas.
[5] Allowable options for canned fish are light tuna, salmon, sardines, and mackerel.

Last updated 10/5/2015

[33] The WIC food packages are referenced from USDA: https://www.fns.usda.gov/wic/wic-food-packages-regulatory-requirements-wic-eligible-foods#FRUITS%20and%20VEGETABLES

Table 23. WIC food Package (b)[34]

SNAPSHOT of the WIC Food Packages [1]

Maximum Monthly Allowances (MMA) of Supplemental Foods For Infants [2]

	Fully Formula Fed (FF)		Partially (Mostly) Breastfed (BF/FF)		Fully Breastfed (BF)	
Foods	Food Packages I-FF & III-FF A: 0-3 months B: 4-5 months	Food Packages II-FF& III-FF 6-11 months	Food Packages I-BF/FF & III- BF/FF A: 0 to 1 month B: 1-3 months C: 4-5 months	Food Packages II-BF/FF & III-BF/FF 6-11 months	Food Package I-BF 0-5 months	Food Package II-BF 6-11 months
WIC Formula	A: 823 fl oz reconstituted liquid concentrate B: 896 fl oz reconstituted liquid concentrate	630 fl. oz. reconstituted liquid concentrate	A: 104 fl. oz. reconstituted powder B: 388 fl oz reconstituted liquid concentrate C: 460 fl. oz. reconstituted liquid concentrate	315 fl. oz. reconstituted liquid concentrate		
Infant cereal		24 oz		24 oz		24 oz
Infant food fruits and vegetables [3]		128 oz		128 oz		256 oz
Infant food meat						77.5 oz

[1] Refer to the full regulation at ***www.fns.usda.gov/wic*** for the complete provisions and requirements for infant formula and infant foods in the WIC food packages.

[2] State agencies must provide at least the full nutrition benefit, as defined in §246.2, to non-breastfed infants.

[3] At State agency option, older infants may be issued a cash-value voucher for fresh fruits and vegetables in lieu of a portion of jarred infant foods.

[34] The WIC food packages are referenced from USDA: https://www.fns.usda.gov/wic/wic-food-packages-regulatory-requirements-wic-eligible-foods#FRUITS%20and%20VEGETABLES

4.3 Decision framework for WIC recipients

4.3.1 Decision Framework

Most economic research explain the participation of WIC based on the traditional cost-benefit framework (Tiehen & Jacknowitz, 2010). For WIC eligible individuals with utility maximization, the participation decision is made when the benefits outweigh the costs with participation. The cost of participation has been mainly focused on two primary fields, stigma and transaction costs (Currie, 2006).

Assistance recipients may feel embarrassed or ashamed of receiving assistance from the Government, especially when the others know. For example, when WIC recipients check out in grocery stores using their food vouchers or EBT card, they may perceive stigma from grocery staff, which may be a strong deterrent to participation for people in need (Yaniv, 1997). As for transaction costs, they include both money and time costs that associated with applying for WIC, following the WIC rules, documenting eligibility and redeeming benefits. In addition, the costs also include the effort and time to initially enroll and renew the benefits. As introduced above, the WIC benefits are a combination of both in-kind benefits (only for fruits and vegetables) and certain amount of food, instead of cash. One of the most significant differences between in-kind benefits and cash transfer is the constraint from in-kind transfer. Basically, there is a fundamental cost of in-kind provision that recipients would always prefer the equivalent value of cash transfer (Lieber and Lockwood, 2018). To redeem WIC benefits, recipients also need to take time and find WIC eligible products.

The redemption process of WIC is more complicated during the time of paper vouchers. WIC recipients need to separate WIC-eligible and non-eligible products and check out in separate lines to present their paper voucher to cashiers. The cashiers would check the eligibility and notify which benefits are redeemed. After transition from paper vouchers to EBT, the WIC recipients only need to scan their EBT card, and the computer program would distinguish the WIC-eligible and non-eligible products (Hanks et al., 2016).

4.3.2 Impact of WIC

As a federal assistance program, one of WIC's primary objectives is to reduce the most common nutrition risk among WIC eligible individuals – insufficient calories. This nutrition risk also strongly correlates with food insecurity (Black et al., 2004; Metallinos et al., 2011; Kreider, Pepper, and Roy, 2016).

WIC's impact on consumption, health, and birth outcomes is widely discussed in the literature. Khan et al., in 2018, find WIC affects participants' consumption pattern by increasing their cereal consumption. Currie and Rajani (2015) use birth records in New York City to find the relationship between WIC and low birth weight reduction. For child outcomes, Chorniy, Currie, and Sonchak in 2018 show that WIC improves child outcomes in various domains, including childhood mental health and grade repetition.

Lots of literature show the positive impact of WIC on consumption, nutrition, and birth outcomes. Oh, Jensen and Rahkovsky (2016) use the difference-in-difference method to estimate the impact of WIC participation, and the impact of 2009 WIC food package change on whole grains' consumption. They confirm that WIC participation is related to more whole grain purchases, and the policy change in 2009 increase this impact. Khan et al., in 2018, also find that WIC affects participants' consumption patterns by increasing their cereal consumption. Generally, low-income households do not consume enough fresh fruits and vegetables, thus, i. Thus, the consumption of these healthy foods is always a public priority for policymakers in the U.S. For children (aged 1-4 years old) in WIC, 128 ounces of fruit juice and an $8 value of voucher or EBT in-kind benefits for fruits and vegetables are provided each month to encourage consumption. Vercammen et al., in 2018 find that comparing with eligible non-participants, WIC participants have significantly more consumption of 100% fruit juice after adjusting children and parents' characteristics.

For pregnancy, health, and non-health outcomes, the positive impacts of WIC benefits on women, infants, and children are confirmed in many studies. Hoynes, Page, and Stevens (2011) use the WIC rollout among counties to control selection bias and confirm that WIC participation positively impacts average birth weight and negatively impacts the fraction of low birth weight. Currie and Rajani in 2015 use a fixed-effect model to investigate the positive impact of WIC on reducing low birth weight in New York City. Rossin-Slater (2013) uses with-ZIP-code variation in WIC clinic openings and closings and maternal fixed effects to show that access to WIC has a positive impact on pregnancy weight gain and birth weight. As for children's health outcomes, Chorniy, Currie, and Sonchak (2018) show that WIC improves child outcomes in various areas, including ADHD, childhood mental health, and grade repetition. Lee and Mackey-

Bilaver in 2007 use sibling fixed-effect models to prove that WIC and SNAP lower the risk of abuse and neglect reports, as well as several nutrition-related illnesses, such as feeding disorder of infancy and early childhood, anemia, and nutritional deficiency. Jackson (2015) also focuses on the non-health effect of WIC. He uses a coarsen exact matching and fixed-effect model to confirm that prenatal and early childhood WIC participation improves cognitive development in the short reading and math learning in the long-term.

4.3.3 BMI for Children and Teens

Body mass index (BMI) is a simple and cheap way to measure body fatness based on height and weight. Though BMI is not diagnostic of body health, it is a convenient rule of thumb to measure how far a person's weight away from normal for a person's height. BMI is calculated from the mass(kilogram) divided by the square of height(meter). For adults older than 20 years old, an individual can be categorized based on BMI range as underweight (BMI under 18.5 kg/m2), normal weight (18.5 to 25), overweight (25 to 30), obese (over 30).

For children (aged 2 to 20), BMI is used differently. Children's BMI is still calculated by weight and height in the same way as adults, but due to the changes in weight, height and their relation to body fatness along with age and development, the BMI is compared with other children at the same age and gender and expressed as a percentile relative to other children. Under the Centers for Disease Control and Prevention (CDC) guideline in the United States, these percentiles are calculated based on CDC growth charts, which were generated from national survey data.[35] Thus, the BMI for a child should be presented and interpreted relative to other children of the same age and gender.

In the United States, the BMI-for-age percentile growth charts are the most recommended measure to assess the weight to height for children and teens. Figure 22 and Figure 23 show the BMI-for-age growth chart for boys and girls aged 2 to 20 separately.[36] With the guideline of CDC, a child or teen (2 years old to 20 years old) can be categorized based on BMI-for-age percentile as underweight (smaller than the 5th percentile), normal or healthy weight (5th percentile to smaller than the 85th percentile), overweight (85th to smaller than the 95th percentile), and obese (equal to or larger than the 95th percentile). Figure24 explains how to interpret a 10-year-old boy's BMI numbers and percentile based on the BMI-for-age growth chart.[37]

---

[35] BMI for child and teen from CDC:
https://www.cdc.gov/healthyweight/assessing/bmi/childrens_bmi/about_childrens_bmi.html
[36] BMI-for-age growth charts are referenced from CDC:
https://www.cdc.gov/growthcharts/data/set1clinical/cj41l023.pdf
https://www.cdc.gov/growthcharts/data/set1clinical/cj41l024.pdf
[37] The example figure is referenced from CDC:
https://www.cdc.gov/healthyweight/assessing/bmi/childrens_bmi/about_childrens_bmi.html

Figure 22. Boys Body Mass Index-for-Age Percentile[38]

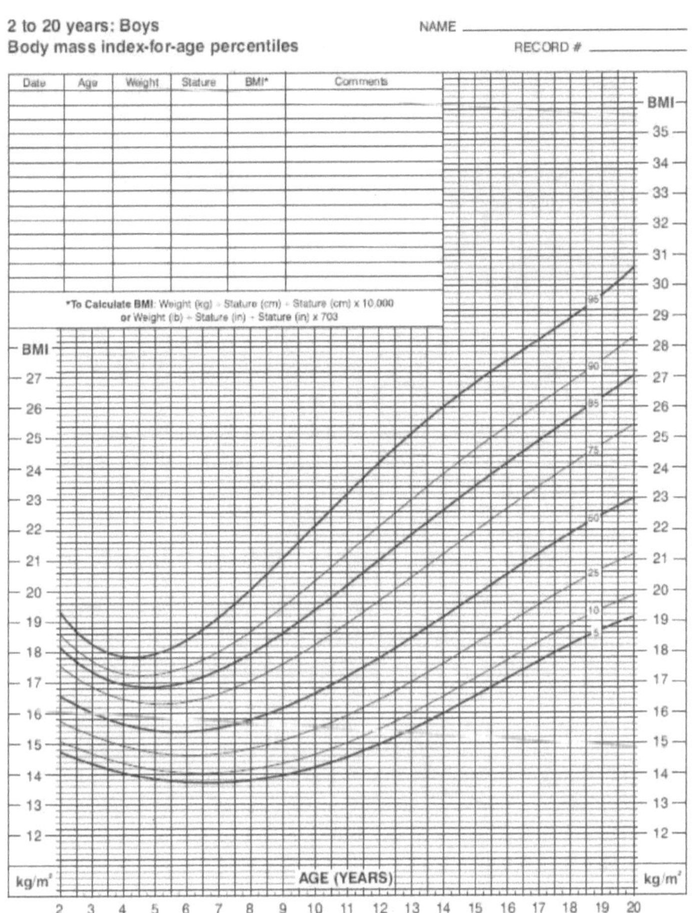

[38] BMI-for-age growth charts are referenced from CDC: https://www.cdc.gov/growthcharts/data/set1clinical/cj41l023.pdf

Figure 23. Girls Body Mass Index-for-Age Percentile[39]

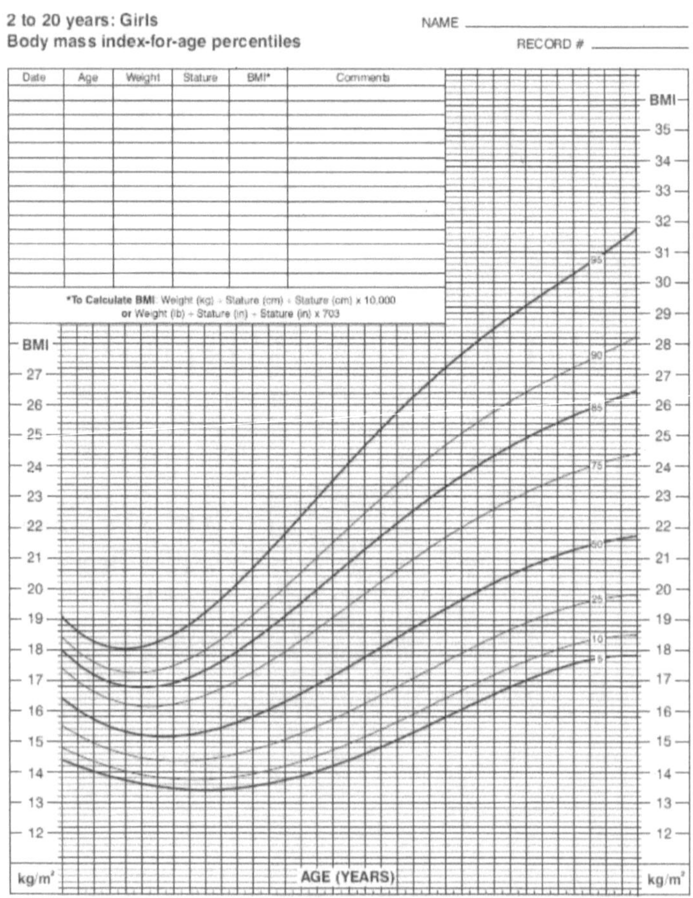

---

39 BMI-for-age growth charts are referenced from CDC: https://www.cdc.gov/growthcharts/data/set1clinical/cj41l024.pdf

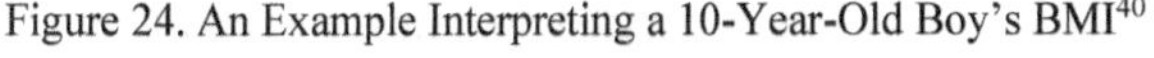

Figure 24. An Example Interpreting a 10-Year-Old Boy's BMI[40]

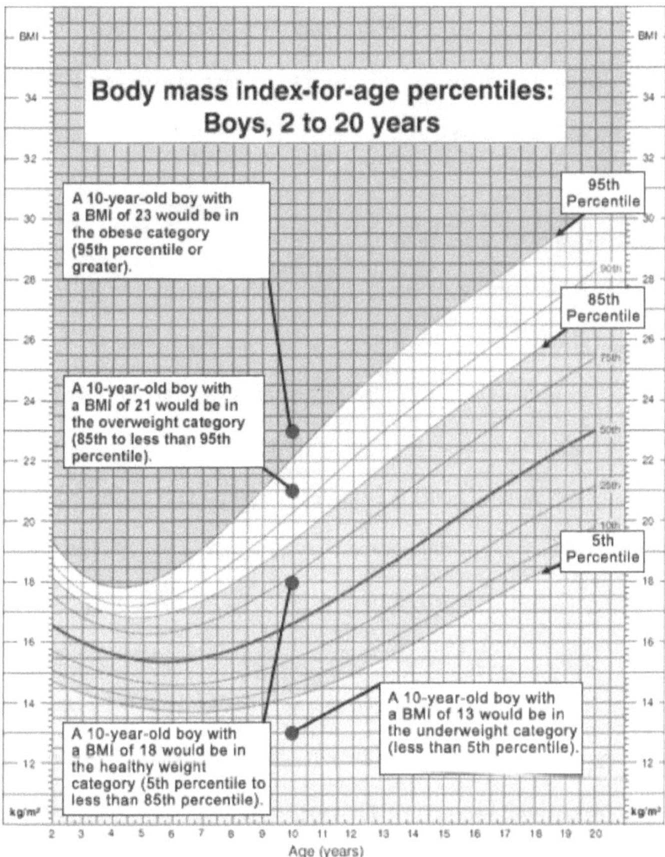

[40] The example figure is referenced from CDC: https://www.cdc.gov/healthyweight/assessing/bmi/childrens_bmi/about_childrens_bmi.html

Similar to BMI for adults, BMI for children and teens is not diagnostic of body health, but an indicator that shows how far a child or teen's weight departs from normal for his or her height, age and gender. It is also a screening tool for potential weight or health problem with children and teens.

4.3.4 Obesity Among Children in WIC

Obesity is associated with various serious health consequences (NIH, 1998), including heart disease, cancer, type2 diabetes, and other health problems that negatively impact life quality (Levi et al., 2012). Obesity also brings a great economic burden because of the high cost of associated diseases (Swinburn et al., 2011). The medical cost of adult obesity in the United States is estimated to be from $147 billion to $210 billion per year, and the direct cost of childhood obesity cost is about $14.1 billion (Levi et al., 2012).

In this work, children and teens overweight is defined as BMI-for-age percentile equal to or larger than 85th percentile, and obesity is defined as BMI-for-age percentile equal to or larger than 95th percentile. Obese children have about twice the risk of dying before 55 compared to children with normal weight (Frank et al., 2010). Overweight and obese children are more likely to have cardiovascular diseases, such as elevated total cholesterol, blood pressure, and insulin (Freedman et al., 2007). They are also at higher risk for other associated diseases, such as asthma (Gilliland et al., 2003), sleeping-disordered breathing (Redline et al., 1999).

Obesity prevalence in the United States is a serious problem, especially among children and teens. Based on a CDC report, for children and teens aged 2 to 19 years old, the obesity prevalence in 2015 -2016 is about 18.5%, and for children aged 2 to 5 years old, the obesity prevalence is about 13.9%. The obesity prevalence is higher among boys aged 2 to 5 years (14.3%) than girls in the same age group (13.5%); however, the difference is not significant (Hales et al., 2017).

Obesity affects more children in low-income households than children in high-income households, and many children in low-income households receive benefits from SNAP and WIC[41] USDA conducts the WIC Participant and Program Characteristics Report (WIC PC) every even year to summarize the characteristics of WIC participants and their weight status. Based on the WIC PC, the obesity prevalence among children aged 2-4 years old in WIC is about 13.9% in 2016 (Pan et al., 2019). In Ohio, the obesity prevalence was about 12.4%, with a 95% Confidence Interval (12.2% to 12.6%) in 2016. Based on the trend analysis in WIC PC, the obesity prevalence in the United States among WIC participants ages 2 to 4 years old is about 14.00% in 2000, increased to 15.5% in 2004, and 15.9% in 2010, and then decreased to 14.5% in 2014. In Ohio, the obesity prevalence increased from 11.6% in 2010 to 12.1% in 2004 and continued to increase to 12.6% in 2010 and 13.1% in 2014. Based on the WIC PC report, Ohio's obesity prevalence from 2010-2016 shows no statistically significant decrease (12.6% in 2010 and 12.4% in 2016) (Pan et al., 2019).

[41] https://www.cdc.gov/obesity/data/obesity-among-WIC-enrolled-young-children.html

4.4 Data

In this chapter, I also use the same administrative data from the Ohio Department of Health WIC, including the WIC participants who receive benefits from March 2015 to February 2019 as Chapter 2. The detailed datasets and variables in the data are introduced in the last chapter.

The datasets I used for this research include participant and participant visit. WIC participants are required to visit the clinic in person at least once every six months, and their health measurements are conducted for both health condition tracking and eligibility. In the participant visit dataset, there are unique participant identifier: participant ID; clinic visit information: visit date, visit type, certification date; health test: weight, height, hemoglobin, hematocrit, risk conditions; participant behavior: smoking, cigarettes per day, drinking, drinking per week, drinking per day, other drugs used, other household smoke; and clinic information: intervention attempted, certified health professional initials. There are unique participant ID, demographic information of participants, the birthdate, participant category, and their certification dates in the participant dataset. The detailed variables in each dataset are shown in the last chapter.

I combine the participant and participant clinic using the unique identifier: participant ID. In this study, since I only consider WIC's length impact on children, only participants with infant and child participant categories are retained. Because I want to investigate the impact of WIC length on health outcomes, participants who only visit the clinic once are excluded (51,965 observations).

The health conditions I investigate are the number of risk conditions and BMI percentile. For each clinic visit in this dataset, 8 variables document the risk condition for participants: Risk Code ID1, Risk Code ID2, Risk Code ID3, … Risk Code ID8. The risk conditions are documented respectively into these 8 variables, from number 1 to number 8. Basically, for each visit, a participant could have at least zero risk conditions and at most eight risk conditions. The risk conditions measured by WIC clinic staff include health measurements (such as at-risk for growth problems, high weight for height, low iron, slow growth, and others); improper behavior (such as an improper bottle of cup use, unhealthy eating habits, unhealthy diet habits, and others). The detailed risk codes and risk conditions are shown in Appendix Table 1. For each visit, I generate the count of risk conditions by counting the number of risk conditions. For the regression analysis of several risks, I include all the infants and children in the dataset.

As for the BMI percentile, the BMI percentile for children needs to calculate based on children's age. I first calculate the age of children when they visit the clinic using the participant dataset's birth date and the visit date from the participant visit dataset. Then I use the BMI calculator[42] from CDC to calculate the BMI percentile for each visit, based on children's weight, height, age, and gender. The BMI percentile only works for children aged from 2 to 20, so for children below 2 years old, I do not calculate their BMI percentile. In the regression analysis for BMI, records when children are smaller than 2, are not included.

---

[42] The calculator is referenced: https://www.cdc.gov/healthyweight/bmi/calculator.html

For WIC's length, I calculate it based on the time length of the first visit date for the participant ID and the visit date. I assume this length demonstrates how many months that a participant keeps receiving WIC benefits. However, a participant might enroll in WIC, drop out, and re-enroll again. In this situation, this participant would have another new participant ID. This participant would be counted twice in my analysis because participant ID is the unique identifier I can use. But this situation should not affect if I use a fixed-effect model. The participant category is also adjusted based on the visit date and birth date; the adjustment is explained in the previous chapter.

4.5 Empirical Approach

To estimate the impact of WIC length on health outcomes, I consider the fixed effect model since I have panel data that documents the number of risks and BMI percentile for every clinic visit. I use the length of months that a child stays in WIC as a source of exogenous variation and determines whether a longer time results in better health outcomes: fewer risk conditions and BMI percentile change. In this way, I try to separate other time-invariant effects on health, such as gender, racial/ethnic, and household demographic conditions.

For the number of risk conditions, since the outcome variable is count with largest 8 and smallest 0, I use a Poisson fixed effect regression. Considering the transition from an infant to a child, which is time-variant, I include a dummy variable that indicates whether this record is for an infant or child. The model is as follows:

$$y_{it} = \beta_0 + \beta_1 Length_{it} + \beta_2 Infant_{it} + \varepsilon_{it}$$

Each y_{it} represents a number of risk conditions for individual *i* in time *t*. The variable infant is an indicator variable that has a value of 0 for child and 1 for infant. The *length* represents how many months the individual *i* in WIC until this clinic visit.

For BMI percentile, I use a regular fixed-effect regression. Since the BMI percentile only works for children aged from 2 to 20, I only calculate BMI percentile for those children, and there is no need to consider the infant indicator in this regression. The model is as following:

$$y_{it} = \beta_0 + \beta_1 Length_{it} + \varepsilon_{it}$$

Each y_{it} represents the BMI percentile for individual *i* in time *t*. The *length* represents how many months the individual *i* in WIC until this clinic visit.

I also conduct a logistic fixed effect model with BMI percentile as a dummy variable: underweight, overweight, and obese. For underweight, it equals 1 when the BMI percentile is less than 5%, and it equals 0 when the BMI percentile is larger or equals to 5% and less than 85%. As for overweight, it equals 1 when the BMI percentile is larger or equals to 85%, and it equals 0 when the BMI percentile is between 5% to 85%. For obese, it equals 1 when the BMI percentile is larger than 95%, and it equals 0 when it is between 5% to 85%.

4.6 Results

4.6.1 Summary Statistics

In Table 24 I presented the top 20 risks that documented in the dataset. Overall, improper bottle or cup use is documented 346,792 times, which is the most frequent risk.

The following most frequent four risks include: baby born to WIC eligible mom, unhealthy diet habits, at risk for growth problem and improper feeding practice.

Table 24. Top 20 Most Frequent Risk Conditions

Risk Condition	Frequency
IMPROPER BOTTLE OR CUP USE	346,792
BABY BORN TO WIC ELIGI MOM	330,445
UNHEALTHY DIET HABITS (CHILDREN)	246,494
BABY BORN TO WIC ELIGIBLE MOM	167,158
AT RISK FOR GROWTH PROBLEMS	144,187
IMPROPER FEEDING PRACTICE	138,652
BREASTFED BY A WIC MOM	131,975
UNHEALTHY DIET HABITS	129,781
UNHEALTHY DIET HABITS (INFANTS)	127,086
BORN EARLY	118,146
HIGH WEIGHT FOR HEIGHT	116,766
IMPROPER INFANT FEEDING	115,701
COND THAT AFFECT NUTRI STAT	106,081
LOW IRON	95,952
LOW BIRTH WEIGHT	81,231
HIGH WEIGHT FOR HEIGHT/AT RISK OF HIGH WEIGHT FOR HEIGHT	77,559
BREASTFED BY A WIC MOM	73,346
BORN EARLY	64,312
SHORT FOR AGE	60,862
SHORT FOR AGE/AT RISK OF SHORT FOR AGE	58,026

In Table 25 I showed the average number of visits and length of WIC and their standard deviation for each individual participant, and the average health conditions when the child firstly visit the clinic and the last time visit. After removing the individuals with only one record (51,965 observations), and with all 0 risk condition (30 observations), there are overall 332,464 individuals in my analysis. On average, an individual visit clinic for about 5.45 times and keeps in WIC for about 24.03 months, which is about 2 years. On average, in the first visit, infants/children in this dataset has about 2.03 risk conditions. And in their last visit, the average number of risk conditions decreases to about 1.62.

As for BMI percentile, after removing records with age under 2 years old, I have totally 148,166 children. Their average BMI percentile in their first visit is about 65.53%, and their average BMI percentile in their last visit increases to about 66.87%.

Table 25. Summary Statistics

Variable	Mean	Std.Dev.		
Number of Visits	5.45	3.38		
Length of WIC (Month)	24.03	18.03		
Observations	332,464			
	First Time Visit		Last Time Visit	
	Mean	Std.Dev.	Mean	Std.Dev.
Number of Risk Conditions	2.03	1.10	1.62	0.89
Observations	332,464			
BMI Percentile	65.53	28.40	66.87	28.34
Observations	194,280			

4.6.2 Main Results

The main regression results are presented in Table 26, 27. In Table 26, Column 1 shows the Poisson fixed effect results of number of risk conditions and Column 2 shows the fixed effect results of BMI percentile. These results indicate that on average, for each additional 10 months in WIC, the number of risk condition decreases about 0.08 for children. The coefficient is statistically significant, which indicates that longer time in WIC reduces the number of risks for WIC infants and children. As for BMI percentile, for each additional 10 months in WIC, the BMI percentile increase about 7.6%. The coefficient is statistically significant, and shows that the longer time in WIC increases the BMI percentile for children age 2 to 5.

Table 26. Main Results (1)

VARIABLES	(1) Risk Count	(2) BMI Percentile
Length of WIC (Month)	-0.00880***	0.0756***
	(6.83e-05)	(0.00195)
Infant	-0.0342***	
	(0.00208)	
Observations	1,813,618	689,771
Number of Participants	332,464	194,280
Individual Fixed Effect	YES	YES

Standard errors in parentheses: *** p<0.01, ** p<0.05, * p<0.1

Table 27, Column 1 shows the logistic fixed effect results of being underweight, Column 2 shows the results for being overweight, and Column 3 shows the fixed effect results of being obese. These three regressions ignore the condition that a WIC participant does not change BMI category during the time of receiving WIC benefits. Thus, for example, the regression in column (1) only includes WIC participants who have turned from underweight to normal weight, or normal weight turn to underweight when they receive WIC benefits. And the results show that, for those WIC children who have changed their BMI category, the longer they stay in WIC, they tend to have worse BMI condition, more likely to be underweight, overweight and obese.

Table 27. Main Results (2)

VARIABLES	(1) Underweight	(2) Overweight	(3) Obese
sincefirstvisit	0.00676***	0.0152***	0.0231***
	(0.00117)	(0.000511)	(0.000628)
Observations	44,391	208,013	147,674
Number of participantid1	8,404	43,960	28,531
Individual Fixed Effect	YES	YES	YES

Standard errors in parentheses: *** $p<0.01$, ** $p<0.05$, * $p<0.1$

4.7 Conclusion and Limitations

In this research, I intend to expand on previous work by exploring the effect of time length that children stay in WIC on their health outcomes: the number of risk conditions and BMI percentile. I use the length of time that a child enrolled in WIC as a source of exogenous variation and determine if those on the program longer do better in health outcomes. I found that longer time in WIC results in fewer risk conditions for infants and children and higher BMI percentile for children. This study's results emphasize the effect of WIC on children's health outcomes and might provide insight into reducing eligible children drop-out. WIC plays an essential role in improving the health of a large number of vulnerable populations. The results of this research could support and encourage WIC enrollment and program utilization. One of the limitations of this study is the subsampling problem of data, which could be solved with the new data from

ODH WIC. And I could also investigate similar questions for pregnant, breastfeeding, and not breastfeeding women in WIC.

Chapter 5. Conclusion

This chapter summarizes the main results, limitations, and future work of my three essays. This book investigates the enrollment and redemption of two main food assistance programs in the U.S., SNAP and WIC.

In the second chapter, I confirm that the rise of SNAP benefits cause SNAP recipients to increase their food-at-home, fruits, vegetable, dairy, and non-alcohol beverage expenditures. Cuts in SNAP benefits led to decreases in expenditures on sweets. Notably, however, the changes in benefits do not significantly impact the allocation of recipients' food expenditure. In other words, expenditure shares did not change.

One of the key limitations of this first study is selection bias. Despite the difference-in-differences and matching methods, I cannot completely resolve select bias. Besides, some of the households in the CES diary survey only provide one week of expenditures. To overcome this, I assume that two weeks of expenditures for these households equals double the amount of one week of expenditures. Third, non-alcohol beverages in this study include water, juice, as well as other sweetened beverages. Expenditure on more narrow product categories, such as sugar-sweetened beverages, could be conducted in future work.

In the third chapter, with the Ohio Department of Health WIC's administrative data, I find a decreasing trend from 2015-2019 in overall enrollment in WIC and redemption of WIC benefits in Ohio. I also confirm that the decreasing trends are not driven by a single participant group or county, or even better economic conditions. This work provides insights that WIC policymakers and service providers can consider in improving program benefits and targeting those who need the program most.

In the fourth chapter, with the same data source as in the third chapter, I find that the length of time enrolled in WIC impacts reducing the number of risk conditions for infants and children and increasing the BMI percentile of children (aged 2 to 5). This chapter's results could provide some insight into the roles that WIC plays in improving children and infant nutrition and health. In future work, a similar analysis could be conducted for women in WIC to show how the length of time they participate may affect their overall health. The data's limitations may exist given the under-sampling problems since the WIC recipients that I do not have are not randomly distributed in the sample. Apart from this, the category of risk conditions in the data could be further investigated, such as only including the health risks or behavior-related risks, and then conducted a similar analysis.

www.ingramcontent.com/pod-product-compliance
Lightning Source LLC
LaVergne TN
LVHW041113150826
845673LV00007B/2039
* 9 7 8 3 3 8 4 2 7 4 3 4 2 *